Megan Steelman's new guide glows with the wisdom she has distilled from her work with thousands of parents-to-be. From firsthand experience, she understands the issues that concern pregnant women and their partners. In this book, she explores these questions and shows her readers the ways to find their own, personal answers."

> —Elmer Grossman, M.D., Clinical Professor of Pediatrics, Emeritus, University of California San Francisco School of Medicine, author of *Everyday Pediatrics and Everyday Pediatrics for Parents.*

Thinking Pregnant is a perfect companion for anyone embarking on the life-altering journey of pregnancy. Megan Steelman offers up-to-date medical information balanced with wisdom and candor. Thinking Pregnant is a must-have for anyone considering having a baby!

> —Kim Mulvihill, M.D., medical reporter for KRON San Francisco, health columnist for Sfgate.com, and the "woman's doc" for Thrive online

Megan Steelman provides a thoughtful examination of the difficulties and joys of the passage into parenthood. This book is an excellent resource for those wishing to enter this stage of life more consciously.

> —Cybele Tomlinson, author of *Simple Yoga* and Director of the Berkeley Yoga Center in Berkeley, California

P THINKING REGNANT

Conceiving
Your New Life
with a Baby

Megan V. Steelman, B.A., A.C.C.E.
Foreword by Rhoda Nussbaum, M.D.

New Harbinger Publications, Inc.

Distributed in the U.S.A. by Publishers Group West; in Canada by Raincoast Books; in Great Britain by Airlift Book Company, Ltd.; in South Africa by Real Books, Ltd.; in Australia by Boobook; and in New Zealand by Tandem Press.

Copyright © 2001 by Megan V. Steelman
                   New Harbinger Publications, Inc.
                   5674 Shattuck Avenue
                   Oakland, CA 94609

Cover design by Amy Shoup
Edited by Lorna Garano
Text design by Tracy Marie Powell

Library of Congress Card Catalog Number: 00-134860
ISBN 1-57224-230-2 Paperback

New Harbinger Publications' Web site address: www.newharbinger.com

03   02   01

10   9   8   7   6   5   4   3   2   1

First printing

With unflagging maternal love I dedicate this book to my children, Austyn Lea Steelman and Laine Sumner Steelman.

Contents

Domestic Violence ❧ The Changing Face of
Friendship ❧ Me, Myself, and I ❧ The
Mother in Me ❧ Like a New Language

Acknowledgments

I owe my biggest debt of gratitude to my sister, Evrith Giovenco, who spent tireless hours combing through my manuscript. Equally important are the many expectant and new parents whom I have taught over the years. Their stories and experiences have been the inspiration for not only much of the book, but have also provided years of fulfillment in my professional life. I also want to thank the following people for their support and feedback: my dedicated editor Lorna Garano and the gracious staff at New Harbinger; my Kaiser support system; Seth Feigenbaum, MPH, M.D.; Rhoda Nussbaum, M.D.; Tanya Wiser, MSW; Maura Varley, MPH, MSW; Sarah Pimental; Vera Grab, R.N.; Brigid McCaw, M.D.; Scott Thomas, Ph.D.; Richard Drumn; my loyal carpool, Nancy Zinn, N.P.; Jenna Lewis, N.P.; and Susan Millar. A big thanks also goes to those who reviewed the manuscript in any one of its many incarnations: Cybele Tomlinson, Laurel Graver, Tandy Parks, Dawn Nakashima, Jonathan Newman, Jim Greenberg, Mary Thomas, Trish Wittmer, Suzie Swanson, Ayn Perry, Sarah Felder, and Devra Noily, and of course my mother Mildred, sister Arla, plus family and friends for seeing me through this project with patience and devotion.

Foreword

It's two A.M. and I can't sleep. My heart and mind are racing too
fast for sleep! You see, I have a son whom I have watched grow
from a black-haired, black-eyed, beautiful baby to a loving,
responsible, and caring young man. He is twenty-two years old
now, and I am enjoying watching him ease into adulthood. He is
more a friend to me than ever.

But this afternoon, after a day of skiing, he and his friend
were driving home with that wonderful feeling of exhaustion,
snaking down the mountain in a river of cars. Not realizing how
tired he was, he shut his eyes and in an instant the car hit a snow
embankment and flipped over, landing on its roof in the middle
of the road. My son is asleep now, safe and unhurt, as is his
friend. They were both wearing seat belts and the car took the
impact without being crushed or crushing them. Yet I can't sleep
because my mind can't stop thinking about how much I love this
wonderful young man. My heart is remembering so many
moments over the last twenty-two years when he filled me with
pride, frustration, intense love, and fear.

Megan Steelman honored me by asking me to write the foreword for her book several months ago. I am an obstetrician/gyne-
cologist and have been in practice for over twenty years in San
Francisco. I also serve as Women's Health Leader for Kaiser Permanente Northern California, an organization that cares for more
than three million members. My professional life has been spent
helping women in their multiple roles as mothers, daughters,
wives, lovers, workers, caregivers, and health care coordinators
for the rest of their families. I have worked with thousands of

women facing the decisions Megan writes about in this book. I have also worked with thousands of women who find themselves pregnant before consciously making the decision to have a baby, an event that will change their lives dramatically. I have been contemplating what I wanted to put into this foreword. As I lay in bed staring at the dark ceiling, thanking God that my son is alive, I realized that this was the time to start writing.

Half of all pregnancies in the United States are unintended, that is, undesired or mistimed. Even when this is not the case, pregnancy, a momentous event, too often occurs before we have asked ourselves the questions Megan addresses in this book. This is not so surprising when you consider how we learn or go about making choices. We begin something new from a state of unconscious incompetence. We are not even aware of what we do not know. As we learn, questions form in our minds. We don't know the answers to the questions at this stage of learning or decision making, but at least we are asking questions. We are now consciously incompetent. As we learn new information and skills, we have to think about what it is we are doing and continue to ask questions. This leads to conscious competence. Finally, when we have learned enough to make the decision or master the skill, we incorporate it into our lives without needing to think about it anymore. We have finished the cycle and are unconsciously competent.

Let's use skiing as an example since it is on my mind this morning! When you first start thinking about becoming a skier, you are in a state of unconscious incompetence. That is, you don't know what you have to learn or what questions to ask. As you begin to talk to other people who have learned to ski, you begin to understand what is involved. Should you rent equipment or buy? Where will you go to learn? Will you go for a week or a weekend? Should you have your friend teach you or take lessons? As you learn more about it, you have more questions to ask. When you started, you didn't even know what you didn't know!

Next, you have enough knowledge and information to know that there is much to learn. Not only do you need to have equipment and instructions, your body needs to learn new skills. You take your first run down the bunny slope and realize that you have to learn to get on and off the lift. Then you have to learn how to turn, how to shift your weight, and how to stop. You realize that there is a lot to learn, and you are conscious of how incompetent you feel at this stage.

With practice and by asking and watching others, you begin to learn and gradually you can ski. You no longer have to think much about getting on and off the lift, even though that caused you great fear before. You can manage the beginner slopes without really thinking about how to move your body. You simply flow down the run. But when you take that first ride down the steeper intermediate slope, you again face your limits. As you reach ever higher skill levels you incorporate your knowledge and accomplish the task with less and less conscious effort.

This same process can apply to parenthood and parenting. Because you are reading this book, I know that you are beyond the first stage of unconscious incompetence. You have consciously chosen to contemplate the questions and issues before your pregnancy or before the birth of your child, and this will give you a leg up on dealing with pregnancy.

The decision to have a baby and how you will handle pregnancy involves many factors. Megan's book gives you a picture of the universe you are entering. She formulates the questions you may not have thought to ask. She provides you with a factual springboard from which you can make decisions on everything from emotional and physical changes to practical considerations like how much it will cost to raise your child. Her book is filled with the wisdom of the thousands of couples she has worked with during her career as a specialist in health education and childbirth preparation. You will see yourself in some of the stories she tells, and in others you will see people whose decisions you will not want to duplicate.

This is a practical and useful guide for women and couples who want to consciously enter into the greatest, most important, most fulfilling, and most challenging experience of life. Dr. Spock helped us know what to do once the baby was in our arms. Megan Steelman helps us know what to think about, ask, and decide before the baby is in our wombs.

My eighty-eight-year-old father tells me that being a parent continues to give pleasure and fulfillment all through life. I know that each day of my children's lives, from the first day I nursed them until today when they are entering adulthood, has been better and better. I continue to learn how to be a better parent. And tonight especially, I know how much they mean to me.

—Rhoda Nussbaum, M.D.
Dorrington, California

Introduction

My hometown of Berkeley, California is also where I went to college. In 1978 I graduated from the University of California Berkeley with what seemed like a useless degree in Social Science. My mother urged me to "just get a B.A., honey; it's a good thing to have." A year later, at age twenty-five, I was newly married, living in Los Angeles, and adrift professionally. Six months later I was among the first in my circle of friends to become pregnant. My daughter, Austyn, would soon change my life forever.

As with most things I do, I jumped into pregnancy and motherhood with very little advance preparation and no lifeboat. My hunger for knowledge and my research skills proved my salvation. The few books available about pregnancy became fixtures on my nightstand. I joined the only prenatal exercise class I could find in Santa Monica. Clothes horse that I am, I did my best to make pregnancy into a fashion statement, which, at the time, was quite a challenge. I absorbed information from whatever sources I could find. Tandy Parks, my fabulous childbirth educator, not only became a great professional inspiration to me, but, after having a child, looked so trim in her Gloria Vanderbilt jeans, she gave me faith that I would once again have a waistline.

My professional journey began in 1982 when I started substitute teaching for a prenatal exercise class at the YWCA in Santa Monica. It was there that I discovered my passion for working with pregnant women and new families. After the birth of my son, Laine, in 1983, I attended the Childbirth Educator Training Program at UCLA and became an American Society of Psychoprophylaxis (ASPO) Certified Childbirth and Breastfeeding

Educator (I needed a B.A. to get into the program, so Mom, as usual, was right). Since then I have taught thousands of pregnant women and their partners, attended numerous births, and developed and implemented training programs for educators and labor doulas (women who provide labor support), along with serving on the faculty of the UCLA Childbirth and Breastfeeding Education training programs, I have been a consultant for a number of pregnancy and labor videos, and have developed visual teaching aids and relaxation cassettes for pregnant and laboring women. My lectures on childbirth and breastfeeding have taken place in various ports of call, including Los Angeles, Berkeley, and Jerusalem. And I have had the opportunity to reach a wider audience with a number of radio and television interviews.

In 1986 after living in Los Angeles for eighteen years, I moved back to my home turf, Berkeley. Currently I am the Director of Perinatal Education and the Breastfeeding Center at Kaiser Permanente in San Francisco, where we have a full range of classes taught in English, Spanish, and Cantonese. I am excited to be branching out into women's health and have co-created *Body in Balance*, an annual series of workshops on women's health offered to the women of San Francisco.

When the opportunity to write a book for women considering pregnancy arose, I jumped at the chance. Writing this book has given me the opportunity to take the past sixteen years of research, professional growth, interaction with students, and education and inspiration from health care professionals and fellow teachers, and craft them into a cohesive body of work. It has also allowed me to reflect on my own experiences of being pregnant at a time when informational doors were just opening. It is fitting that this project has taken nine months from start to finish.

In reading this book, I encourage you to use it in the way that best suits your needs. You might want a cover-to-cover experience, or to use it more as a resource guide and plunge directly into the chapter that is of interest to you at the moment. You will find a worksheet at the end of each chapter. This is designed to help you focus on the information that is most relevant to you and give you a springboard for thinking about various issues and talking with your partner and other loved ones about your hopes and concerns.

When preparing pregnant women for labor, one of my standard tidbits of anxiety-reducing wisdom is: "Breathe in, breathe out, take each contraction as it comes, and stay in the moment." Apply this wisdom to your own life as you begin to "think pregnant." Your childbearing years are a spectacular time of life—a time when you are engaged in a very dynamic rapport with yourself and those around you. As you move toward motherhood, keep your sense of humor, fill your days with laughter and love, and live each vital moment to its fullest.

—Megan V. Steelman
Berkeley, California

1

How Ready Are You?

Of all the decisions you will make in your adult life, deciding to become a parent is perhaps the most overwhelming. You are making a commitment not just to yourself, but also to another human being who will be dependent on you. In other aspects of your life, both large and small, you are accustomed to having options. You accept a job, it doesn't work out, you quit and find a new one. You move into a new neighborhood and find you aren't comfortable there, you move. You enter into a friendship or relationship that doesn't work out, you move on. But bringing a child into the world requires an unending commitment. You become pregnant and give birth and, boom, you fall in love in a way you never thought possible and there you are, committed for life. This involves not just the awesome responsibility, but the unavoidable emotional highs and lows that go along with being a parent. Buckle up: You're in for quite a ride!

The Pregnancy Decision

The pregnancy decision is more complex for women today than it was for previous generations. Women's roles and priorities have changed significantly and many of them are delaying the decision until their mid-thirties and early forties. Some women don't find themselves in a solid, future-bound relationship until then; others agonize for years until they feel 100 percent certain about their decision. Sometimes a woman is ready and her partner isn't, or vice versa. Many women have educational and or career goals they want to achieve prior to committing themselves to parenthood. Most people have an ideal financial state they want to reach before taking on the responsibility of children. Women have concerns that if they do have a baby, it will threaten their freedom, the beauty of their bodies, or the careers they have worked so hard to build. Overall, there is an enormous fear for many women that by becoming "mother" they will lose their identity.

> *From her late twenties to mid-thirties, Margaret, an artist and an athlete, had an on-again, off-again relationship with her boyfriend, who was five years older than she. They dated and broke up numerous times until they decided to get married when she was thirty-three. She continued to be involved in local sports and the art community and returned to school to earn her MFA. By age thirty-four, she knew she was going to have to face the pregnancy decision sooner rather than later. She knew she wanted to be a mother, but felt concerned that her independence and creativity would be stifled by it. Soon after graduating she became pregnant, and though it was not exactly a surprise, it still brought up many conflicting feelings for her about her identity and her life path. Who would she become once she had a child?*

When a woman's biological clock is ticking at a furious pace, she may make what seems like a rash decision to nab the nearest man or visit the closest sperm bank to get pregnant. Her vision of the perfect life partner is replaced by the urgency of her maternal impulse.

> *When Clara was in her thirties she lived with a man who was almost twenty years her senior and had already had a family. Whenever the subject of children came up, he would say, "You don't want to be a mother—it's too much work." He made it very clear that he had no intention of having more children. Their relationship ended when she was forty, at which point she realized she had sacrificed her desire to have children to it. In the hopes of finding someone with whom she could have children, Clara spent a year meeting men through personal ads, but found no one suitable. At age forty-three she decided to have a baby on her own by utilizing the services of a sperm bank.*

There is still a lot of pressure in our society for women to become mothers in order to feel complete. But indeed, there are women who search their souls and come to the conclusion that parenthood just isn't for them. This decision, based on a number of factors, can be painful for some, a relief for others. The hardest part may be breaking the news to their own parents who have been eagerly awaiting grandchildren.

Am I Ready?

When making a conscious decision to become pregnant, a number of "Am I Ready" questions are bound to pop up. You may already be asking yourself some or all of the following:

* Am I ready emotionally, financially, and physically to be a parent?

* Am I ready age-wise to be thinking about parenthood?

* Am I ready to balance my career with the demands of parenting?

* Am I ready for my body to change dramatically?

* Am I ready to deal with the stress if I don't become pregnant immediately?

* Am I ready to change or strengthen my relationship so it will survive the stress of caring for a new baby?

* Am I ready to endure labor?

* Am I ready to handle the new identity that comes with being a mom?

* Am I ready to tap into the stamina I know I will need?

* Am I ready to provide a child with as much love as he or she will need to grow up well adjusted?

* Am I ready to shift the focus of my world to my child?

You may read through these questions and find yourself answering "no" more then "yes," or you may become aware that you are in a state of ambivalence about the prospect of becoming a mother. Doubt, when on the verge of a decision that has such an impact on your physical, emotional, spiritual, and financial life, is normal. Even women who design their lives with the goal of pregnancy in mind have fleeting moments in which they wonder, "Is this really what I want to do?" "Am I sure I want to change my life to this degree?" "Maybe I should wait another year and then think about it."

When it comes to facing the unknown, most of us do so with more than a little trepidation.

On the other hand, you may have answered "yes" to all these questions, feeling that you are prepared and eager to have a baby.

However the cards fall for you as you think about your life plans, remember that knowledge goes a long way in allaying the fear of the unknown.

The Sifting Process

As you consider parenthood and think about how you were parented, you are likely to find that there are things your parents did that you do not want to repeat with your child. Even if you feel your parents treated you fairly and with respect, you will probably vow that you will never do or say certain things. This process of sifting out the behaviors you'd like to repeat from the ones you wouldn't will help you become a more conscious, compassionate mother. You may, however, find it challenging to resist the temptation of replicating those behaviors once you have children!

"I'll Never Do to My Children What My Parents Did to Me"

All parents have pet phrases that they use repeatedly with their children. Phrases like:

❋ "If you think I'm fooling just try me and see."

❋ "I'll thank you to keep a civil tongue in your mouth, young lady."

❋ "If you don't have anything nice to say, don't say anything at all."

❋ *"Why?* Because I'm the mother."

❊ "When you're eighteen you can do it however you want, but as long as you're living under *my* roof you'll do it my way."

Certainly you can add to this list of phrases that make you cringe every time you hear them, after which you'll swear never to act like your parents. Many of us grow up thinking we can avoid the pitfalls of acting as they did and have total confidence that we will do a better job when we have kids of our own. The parenting practices we don't want to repeat run the gamut.

Molly's mother had no respect for her daughter's privacy. She couldn't keep a secret and would freely divulge details about her daughter's personal life to friends and neighbors. For Molly, becoming a trustworthy mother was her greatest aspiration.

Elena's mother was a political activist, always involved in someone else's cause. Elena swore that when she became a mom her cause would be her children.

Then of course there are the things we admire in our parents, the things we want to emulate once we have children.

Aviva's mother went against the grain in the fifties and didn't toilet train her children until they were ready to initiate it on their own. Even with all the disapproving stares and comments, Aviva's mother stuck to her personal philosophy, feeling it was in the best interest of her children. When Aviva had her own children and researched various opinions about potty training, her respect for her mother grew as she chose to follow in her footsteps.

The process of sifting out the positive tactics that our parents used from those that we don't want to repeat shouldn't be taken lightly. What are the family behavior patterns, communication styles, rituals, traditions that you want to preserve? What are those that you would not care to continue? Make a list. Encourage your partner to make a list. Talk about these issues before becoming pregnant. Part of being a conscious parent is moving away from the complacent attitude that says, "This is the way it has always been done" and toward one that says, "This is how we will choose to do it."

Becoming a parent is like having a huge mirror stuck in front of your face. We seem to be able to run from our past until we have children. Once we are parents our own childhood zooms into view and issues come up that we can't bypass. We ask questions like:

* ❊ What will I do differently?

* ❊ What did I appreciate about my upbringing that I would like to incorporate into my own parenting techniques?

* ❊ Do I want to discipline my children the way I was disciplined? If not what will I do differently?

* ❊ What type of role model do I want to be?

* ❊ In what religion will I raise my child?

Some of the choices you make will be easy; others will be a struggle. Your parents may find your new values threatening, or they may be extremely supportive of the decisions you make.

That Lady in the Magazine

We've all seen her. You know, the one on the back cover of the baby magazine you've picked up at your gynecologist's office. She's wearing a white, floor-length robe adorned with lace, her hair is sleek and perfectly cut, lips and cheeks shiny and glowing. She has an air of elegance and relaxation that eludes you even under the best of circumstances—and she's holding a new baby. Her picture conjures up images of spotless kitchens, gleaming toilets, fragrant baskets of folded laundry, and of course, dinner in the oven. She may not be your exact fantasy of new motherhood, but let's face it, we all have one.

We create an ideal image of our future role as a mom often without even being aware that our vision is unrealistic, and these images play into how well we cope with reality when it rears its imperfect head. It can be so dreamy to think of yourself as a new mommy, surrounded by the new baby smell, cuddling a warm, soft, tiny body and feeling fulfilled. At times it is all those things and more, but between these dreamy lines there are pages of text that we often can't see in advance—as if there is some enormous curve in the road ahead that is beyond our vision.

A period of innocence usually prevails before life as you know it becomes something you could never have imagined. That is precisely the point here: You can never imagine just how much your life will change until you gain firsthand experience. A prevailing sentiment among seasoned parents when in the company of a pregnant woman is, "She doesn't know what she's in for." The reality is that your life will be turned upside down and inside out in a way that you never dreamed possible.

This is not to suggest that having a baby will make your life worse; it will simply never be the same. You will have a "new normal" in your life. You will acclimate to your new identity and all its implications, and will most likely find that the day-to-day life of being a mother is far different from what you had once pictured. In many ways your life will be richer, deeper, and more fulfilling. A day will arrive when you'll find yourself thinking, "What did I do with my time before I had my baby?"

The New Normal

A new mom I once worked with observed that her husband often prefaced statements with, "When things return to normal . . ." It was a rude awakening when he realized that "normal" was a thing of the past, that a "new normal" was already in place.

Here are some things that will change in your life:

✻ You will be sleep deprived for a period of months, perhaps even years.

✻ You may feel so much love for your baby that it will eclipse any other love you feel.

✻ Your relationship with your partner will feel stressed for a period of time, though going through pregnancy, birth, and parenting together often strengthens the bond between parents.

✻ You may find in the years to come that spontaneous sex will be hard to come by (but you'll be too tired to care!).

✻ Your emotions may seem like out-of-town guests whom you've never met before and don't really like.

✻ You may find yourself not living up to the image of ideal motherhood you've created.

✻ Your body may seem unrecognizable.

❧   Your breasts will not belong to you for some time if you breast-feed (or to your partner, for that matter).

It's hard to imagine how one small baby can cause such huge changes in your life. Pediatricians, when they schedule your first postpartum appointment, allow for extra time because they know what a drama it is the first time you leave the house with a newborn. Simple tasks take twice as long as before, and scheduling pretty much goes out the window for at least the first two months. You will more than likely have at least one day when you are still in your robe at five in the evening.

At four-thirty Beatrice and her three-week-old daughter, Mona, settled down on the couch for what she hoped would be an afternoon nap when the phone rang. It was Bea's coworker, Robyn, calling from work. When Bea asked her how she was, she chirped, "Oh, I have had quite the day, Bea. I had a huge meeting with all the managers on the team at nine this morning and Doris asked me to head the new environmental task force, you know the one you got off the ground. We had lunch at that fabulous new Italian restaurant downtown, and this afternoon I gave the presentation I've been working on for the past month—Doris wants to use it at the regional conference! Enough about me and my boring life. What about you and my darling Mona? How are my girls?" Bea opened her mouth to answer and burst into tears, realizing that all she had done that day was feed Mona, burp Mona, bathe Mona, and change Mona's diapers. Here it was almost five in the evening and she was still in her robe, unshowered, and had accomplished virtually nothing all day.

Overachievers beware! Time and accomplishment take on a whole new meaning during the early weeks of motherhood. In fact, Beatrice had accomplished a lot as a new mother. She had done exactly what her baby needed. If you are a list maker, used to devising long lists each day and systematically crossing items off of them, be prepared for a shock.

When Laura got pregnant with her first child, her mother, who had raised five children, warned her that she would not be cruising through her lists once the baby came. After the baby arrived, her mother's advice was: "Make a list of one thing every day. If you accomplish that one thing, feel great. One *thing means one thank-you note, one phone call, one load of laundry, or even a shower."* At two months postpartum, Laura, a dynamic Los Angeles lawyer and compulsive list maker, said it was the best advice she'd received. It made a huge difference in her adjustment to motherhood. She was sure to let her mother know how much she appreciated it.*

Organization is really the key to keeping your head above water as a new mother, but keep in mind that it will probably take at least two months before establishing any semblance of order in your home. Until then, sleep, not organization, will be your main priority. It might feel as if life will never run smoothly again. Give yourself time to get your bearings as a new mother; it is definitely a process.

Spontaneity in your relationship pretty much becomes a distant memory for about the next eighteen years. Dinners, movies, outings of any kind, and lovemaking all have to be planned. You may end up taking the baby with you for the first several years until you feel ready to separate. Your desire for outside entertainment diminishes significantly. Who needs it anyway? Your baby is the best entertainment in town. As one new parent said, "We've had our life—been to the theatre, the opera, traveled, had many opportunities. We're ready to stay home with our baby."

". . . Not My Life"

For some of us, the very thought of these changes feels threatening. It's a huge adjustment to rearrange your life and priorities around your baby's needs. You might find yourself wondering, "Will I have a life anymore?" Some women refuse to believe that a baby will change their lives or their emotional state.

Norma was a dedicated career woman, who in no way was going to let either her hormones or motherhood change her life. When her baby was two months old her childbirth educator called her to check in. Here is her unedited response: "This experience is off the charts. It's like I'm breathing different air." When asked about her work, which had been so important to her, she replied, "I could give a flying fuck about my career. People in my office know that if they need anything from me, they'd better get it on my desk by four o'clock because I am out of here by five on the dot."

The Grandparents

Your relationship with your parents will certainly take on a different tone. In becoming a mother you truly become an adult in the eyes of your parents. It may be challenging when you begin to assert your role as a mom, particularly if you and your parents have different philosophies regarding child rearing.

In this era we are encouraged to respond to our babies very differently from what many of our mothers were taught. Many pediatricians encourage parents to respond to a crying baby in a spontaneous rather than structured way. Demand feeding is considered better for the baby than scheduled feeding. We are taught that you can't spoil a baby under six months of age because they don't yet understand cause and effect, e.g., if I cry, that wonderful lady with the warm milk will come pick me up and feed me. We are encouraged to give breast milk, not formula to our babies for at least the first year of life. This is a dramatic departure from the way some of us were raised, and it isn't uncommon for grandparents to feel out of the loop regarding the parenting values of their children's generation.

When Your Buttons Are Pushed

It is inevitable that grandparents will do certain things with your baby and growing child that go against the grain of your parenting ideals. Now is the time to begin thinking about how you will respond to this.

* What will you do if your mother gives a pacifier to your newborn and you are a "no pacifier" purist?

* What if your father-in-law takes it upon himself to bathe your week-old baby and you feel he's overstepping his grandparental boundaries?

* What if your mother-in-law serves sugar- and fat-laden foods to your child when you are trying to raise him on a more wholesome diet?

* What if your father bribes your child to eat dinner by offering her dessert first?

We all have our buttons that get pushed and these little things can feel enormous to a new, anxious parent. The truth is, most of the things grandparents do are relatively harmless, if they're done with love and positive intention. Children learn quickly that there are different rules with different people and as long as you feel your parents or in-laws are respecting your basic parenting values, it is wise to let go of the small things. A brief stint with grandparents will not undo what you accomplish with consistent parenting. If your child's grandparents will be involved with your child on a regular basis, it can't hurt to start educating them now. Give them books on parenting and take them to classes as you begin to educate yourself.

Never Say Never

You had dinner with them again last week, your friends with the new baby. You know, the ones you had weekly dinner and movie dates with, the ones who went backpacking with you on weekends, the ones who went wine tasting in the Napa Valley with you just a year ago. The friends who now talk exclusively about the following topics: how many times the baby woke up last night, how many times the baby pooped during the day, how many hours the baby napped. You politely decline a third chance to watch the labor video, and *ooh* and *aah* over baby photos that were taken yesterday and developed at the one-hour processing lab today. Getting into bed later that night, you and your partner give each other a knowing look, which, without words, says, "We will never be like them." *Never*, especially when said in reference to parenthood, is a dangerous word. You too will find the details of your baby's daily life to be of unparalleled interest. Some things are simply inevitable.

Friendships change once you become parents. Many of your nonparent friends will lose patience with your obsession, just as you have lost patience with new-parent friends. You will seek out other mothers because they are going through the same things you are and they are the ones who will have the stamina for detailed baby poop conversations. Your world will revolve around your child and your interests will change. You will make new "mom" friends—in the park, in your neighborhood, at parent-infant groups, infant massage classes, the grocery store. These new friends might not be the type of people you normally gravitate toward, but the fact that you have babies the same age creates an instant bond.

There will often be one or two friends who will enthusiastically take on the role of surrogate aunt or uncle and hang in there with you and your child through sickness and health. They will baby-sit for you, maybe on a regular basis, and show authentic interest in the growth and development of your child. Cherish these people. Keep in mind that some of them will be parents in the future and you will become a guru dispensing invaluable parenting advice to them.

Changing Lives, Changing Bodies

One thing is unavoidable during pregnancy: Your body will change. Some women take this in stride, while others feel betrayed when they can no longer fit into their favorite pair of jeans. You will most likely experience a combination of feelings as your belly pops out and friends and strangers react to your new figure. People, by the way, are not always tactful and often come with their own agendas.

> *Mara was so excited and full of questions about her changing body. She wanted to share her experience with other women. In her third month, still slim and barely showing, she joined a prenatal exercise class. She was hoping not only to learn some new exercises but to also find a supportive group of women. Instead of the warm welcome she anticipated, they all glared at her because she didn't look pregnant.*

> *Susan was somewhat shy and uncomfortable with her changing body. When people singled her out in public it made her even more self-conscious. She couldn't get used to people stopping her in the market and saying things like, "You are so huge!" or "You look like you are due any minute." She also became fed up with hearing other women's horror stories about their labor.*

As you get bigger and enter your third trimester, don't be surprised if strangers approach you and say things like, "You must be having twins!" "My God, you are huge, are you due next week?" Pregnant women are like magnets for these comments. It isn't enough that you are going through a host of psychological and physical changes; you also become the automatic recipient of unsolicited advice and observations. Shopkeepers, waitresses, and passersby on the street put their hands on your belly without even asking and say things like, "I can tell from the way you are carrying from side to side that this is a girl, and I'm never wrong." "This is a boy because you are all out in front, like a train."

Self-Image

For better or worse, a woman's self-image is often strongly connected to her body. We self-identify by our dress size, waist size, and our particular style of dress. Even if a woman yo-yos in weight and dress size, the physical changes of pregnancy can threaten her self-image. For some women the hardest transition is when they can no longer button their jeans. For others it is when they can no longer tuck in their shirt. And for still others it is when they can no longer see their toes.

Some women feel unattractive during pregnancy, even if they get feedback to the contrary from their partner, friends, or coworkers. Some feel uncharacteristically beautiful and full of life. Women's feelings about their bodies during pregnancy are highly particular.

In the beginning before you are officially showing, it is almost impossible to wrap your mind around how much your body will change. If you find out early, it may be three, four, or even six months before you show. Then once you start showing, each day will bring new feelings, the most prevalent one being disbelief at the proportions your body is achieving. The amazing thing is that you continue to grow. By the third trimester you may have outgrown your early maternity wardrobe and need to buy new clothes.

The good news is that maternity clothes are more stylish than ever. Pregnant women are no longer stuck with the limited choice and unsophisticated styles that their mothers had to endure. A number of designers are making fashionable, elegant clothing, which certainly help to preserve a feeling of attractiveness.

The Mechanics of Maneuvering

Spatial relations and maneuvering through tight spaces can become quite tricky as your body changes. Some women find it difficult to accept that they can no longer do all the things they could in their prepregnancy days.

Leslie parked in the hospital lot on her way to her childbirth education class. Getting out, she tried to slip between her car and the one parked next to her and realized, after turning her body to the right and to the left, that she couldn't fit between the side mirrors. Her startled expression reflected her realization that her body had drastically changed.

Practice Makes Perfect

In high school sex education classes they now encourage teens to experience the responsibility of parenthood by giving them a "baby" for a week. This baby sometimes comes in the form of a sack of flour, other times as a raw egg. Some even use high-tech dolls that need to be fed, changed, and tended to at regular intervals. The teenager's job is to know where the baby is at all times, making sure someone is caring for it if they go out. It is an eye-opener for young, carefree people to have this kind of responsibility even for a week. They need to take the baby to football games, parties, dances, and other social events.

You probably won't want to carry a raw egg around with you in your leather handbag, but if you are an animal lover you may want to get a pet and practice being a caretaker, setting limits, and nurturing a dependent in a consistent way. It might help increase your confidence and get you ready for parenting. Just remember that this pet will be child number one and will most likely become jealous when the baby arrives! On the other hand, it may be more practical for you to spend more time with your niece, nephew, or friend's baby. This is a great way to gain valuable parenting experience. There is nothing like feeding, changing, and comforting the real thing. And, of course, when it isn't yours, you can give it back.

The Ride of Your Life

Let's face it, no matter how prepared you think you are, becoming a mother will look and feel like nothing you have ever done in your life. You can anticipate an unparalleled number of changes in your feelings, your body, your relationships, and your identity. One new mother said she felt like she'd read the book that was designed to prepare her for motherhood, but that it was in a language she didn't understand. She was in no way prepared for the intensity of the new emotions that surfaced once her baby was born. The key message here is: Be prepared for the ride of your life.

How Ready Are You? Worksheet

When I consider whether or not I am ready for motherhood, I feel:

☐ Prepared

☐ Unprepared

Because:

When I consider whether or not I am ready for the physical changes of pregnancy, I feel:

☐ Prepared

☐ Unprepared

Because:

When I wonder if I can become the kind of mother I want to be, I feel:

☐ Prepared

☐ Unprepared

Because:

When I consider how much my relationship with my parents and parents-in-law might change, I feel:

☐ Prepared

☐ Unprepared

Because:

2

Making a Baby

We all learned about the mechanics of sex and baby making during adolescence, but how many of us really understand the biological dynamics of pregnancy? Do you know when you are ovulating and most fertile? When you're not fertile? When to make love to maximize the chances of becoming pregnant?

Ovulation

Here is a quick refresher on how ovulation works. In normal circumstances, fourteen days prior to the onset of your period your ovary releases an egg. If the egg is not fertilized, the lining of the uterus sheds, resulting in a menstrual period.

Your Most Fertile Time

In order to conceive you need to have intercourse around the time of ovulation; your most fertile time is from twenty-four to thirty-six hours prior to the release of the egg. Some women have predictable menstrual cycles and ovulate right on schedule every month. These women obviously have an easier time knowing when they are the most fertile. Some can tell when they are ovulating because they get a particular type of lower backache and experience a watery discharge. Other women's reproductive cycles seem to have a mind of their own, and planning conception is nearly impossible.

More and more women are using urine ovulation prediction kits. Although sometimes hard to read, when these home urine test kits turn positive there is approximately a 90 percent chance that ovulation will take place in the next twenty-four hours. A woman's basal body temperature is slightly elevated when ovulating and the cervical mucus (called "fertile mucus") is thicker. Some women do a temperature check every morning as well as check the consistency of their mucus. As mentioned, a woman's most fertile period is from twenty-four to thirty-six hours prior to ovulation, but she can conceive eighteen and possibly up to twenty-four hours following the release of the egg. The life span of a freshly ovulated egg is twelve to twenty-four hours. Sperm can live two to three days in a woman's cervical mucus. Even when a woman puts this knowledge into practice, it can still take some time to conceive.

When Can I Start?

A question you might be pondering is: "When can I start trying to conceive?" For a healthy woman with no previous history of substance use, who is not significantly overweight, and not on a birth control method that impacts fertility, the answer is "Right now!" Although one exception to this is if you have had a rubella vaccine recently. You are advised to wait three months to give the body time to process and eliminate the virus. If you are not vaccinated and you were to contract rubella it could cause birth defects including deafness, encephalitis, and heart problems.

If You've Been Using Birth Control

Once you discontinue using birth control the amount of time you will need to wait before having unprotected sex will vary. In the meantime using a barrier method of birth control (condom, diaphragm, cervical cap) may be recommended. Certain types affect fertility, others don't. For more detailed information or if you have personal concerns, contact your medical care provider.

How Long Will It Take?

Certainly the younger you are when you begin trying, the better the chance that you will become pregnant quickly. If you are not racing against the clock, enjoy yourself. Relax and enjoy making love with your partner without having to worry about birth control. Try not to over focus on "we are trying to make a baby." Who knows, you may become pregnant the first time, but if you don't, you can try again next month. A sense of trust and faith are great allies. Remember: You are not in the driver's seat on this one. Toby and Ramona, both trying to become pregnant, had very different approaches.

> *Toby was twenty-eight when she first began considering pregnancy. For both her sister-in-law and her best friend it had taken some time to conceive, so she knew from the outset that it might take a while. She decided that a "no pressure" attitude would serve her best. She gave herself a year grace period. Instead of being anxious about the outcome, Toby's attitude allowed her and her partner to enjoy each moment together. After nine months she became pregnant.*

> *At age thirty-four Ramona felt that she had no time to lose and was determined to become pregnant. She diligently checked her temperature every morning and made love with her husband, Kenny, as often as possible when she was ovulating. She thought about pregnancy constantly and read every book she could find. The arrival of her period each month would trigger a deep depression. In addition, her desire to have a baby now was putting a great deal of strain on her relationship with Kenny. Lovemaking was becoming stressful for both of them. After six months she decided it was time for medical intervention and sought the counsel of a fertility specialist. Tests revealed that Kenny had slow-moving sperm. The first thing they tried was insemination, hoping that if the sperm were injected into the uterus, bypassing the cervix it would have a better chance of making it to the egg. After three inseminations, many tears, and a significant amount of strain on both her marriage and her own emotional well-being, Ramona became pregnant.*

Setting Realistic Timeframes

Regardless of your age, it can take longer than anticipated to become pregnant so you always want to give yourself a realistic window of time. Remember that conception rates decrease with age.

* ❈   At age twenty-five the chances of conception with each ovulation are approximately 25 percent.

* ❈   At age thirty the chances are 20 percent.

* ❈   At age thirty-five the chances are 12–15 percent.

* ❈   At age forty the likelihood drops dramatically to 7 percent each month.

It Can Seem Like a Miracle

It often appears that there is no rhyme or reason to when a woman conceives. Some women with no intention of conceiving get pregnant; others who want desperately to become pregnant try and try with no results. When you really think about conception and all the factors that need to be in place at once, it can seem more like a miracle than a physiological occurrence. We have all heard stories about women whose odds of conceiving were slim to none and still became pregnant. Some women report that once they stopped striving to conceive they became pregnant.

What Can I Do To Increase My Chances?

Care providers vary in their approach but most feel that after three to six months of unsuccessful attempts it's time to get a little more serious and consider your options. If you are in your thirties and feeling pressed for time you might not want to wait the full six months before coming up with a plan. Discuss your eagerness and concerns with your care provider. If you are in your forties and have been trying for a year you might be advised to consider in vitro fertilization (IVF) at the very first doctor's visit.

There are many new theories about what women can do to increase the chances of conception. Though some may sound far-fetched, studies are currently being conducted to determine the impact of a wide range of factors on conception. Be sure to speak with your medical care provider before trying any of them. Perhaps you have heard of some of the following.

Cough Syrup

Some anecdotal evidence suggests that taking two tablespoons of Robitussin cough syrup in the two to three days before ovulation can increase your chances of conceiving. It is suspected that the active ingredient in this over-the-counter medicine changes the cervical mucus, allowing sperm to bypass it more readily. Before trying this be sure to discuss it with your physician.

Prayer and Relaxation

In recent years some researchers have begun to study the impact of prayer and relaxation on conception. Some suspect that this may increase the chances of pregnancy for certain women.

Frequent Intercourse Around Ovulation

Numerous studies conducted cross-culturally have shown that couples who have intercourse more frequently around ovulation have a higher monthly conception rate than couples who make love only once or twice throughout this time. Three times during the week of ovulation is optimal.

Alternative Methods

There are various herbal and homeopathic recommendations for boosting fertility. Alternative medicine providers such as naturopaths, osteopaths, herbalists, acupuncturists, and homeopathic healers typically offer these. It is important to check with your health care provider before trying any of these methods.

Fertility Counseling

If conception does not occur within a given window of time, which will vary from woman to woman depending on her age and health history, her care provider will recommend a fertility workup to try to identify why conception is not taking place. Depending on your history, there are a variety of diagnostic tests that can be performed. These tests will be directed at examining your reproductive anatomy, your ovulation, and the condition of your eggs. Some of the conditions these tests look for are:

❋   Blocked fallopian tubes

❋   Uterine fibroids, ovarian cysts, or endometriosis

❋   Abnormal hormone levels

❋   Anovulation (lack of ovulation)

Your partner's sperm count will be checked as well. About half of the time, infertility is caused by male factors. Testing of the sperm can indicate how quickly the sperm moves, or if the count is so low that fertilization is unlikely to occur. Artificial insemination might be advised in the hopes of maximizing motility and quality of the sperm.

If you have a history of three or more pregnancy losses there may be hormonal, chromosomal, or immunologic reasons why you aren't able to carry a pregnancy. Certain medications as well as bed rest throughout the first trimester might be indicated. Treatment directed at a specific abnormality discovered during testing can be quite successful. Unfortunately, testing is able to pinpoint an abnormality in only a minority of couples with multiple miscarriages.

A Word about In-Home Pregnancy Testing

The use of in-home pregnancy tests has become widespread in the past fifteen to twenty years. If they are used according to directions, these tests are about 85 to 95 percent accurate, though the accuracy rates vary among the different manufacturers. Also, the false negative rate decreases substantially if you wait until at least two weeks following ovulation to use it. What this means is that a woman can discover that she is pregnant as early as two weeks after ovulation. The positive aspect of this is that it gives you early access to information that will help you evaluate your situation. If you know that you are pregnant early on, then from the outset you can be diligent about your health and the health of your baby. However, not all pregnancies are viable. In fact, at least 15 percent of those that occur in women in their twenties end in miscarriage, and this rate increases with age. At least half of all miscarriages are due to chromosomal abnormalities in the developing embryo. Prior to in-home testing, an early miscarriage (called a blighted ovum) may never have been detected; a woman simply would have experienced a heavier period.

Now that we are able to learn about and attach to a pregnancy so readily, an early miscarriage can be traumatic. The grief associated with miscarriage, particularly an early one, is for the most part overlooked. People generally think, "It wasn't a real baby, so it must not be too bad," or "She'll become pregnant again and everything will be fine." In fact, a miscarriage is a legitimate loss for both a woman and her partner and they need grieving time. There are more and more books being written on the subject of miscarriage. Women and their partners find solace in support groups, journaling, talking, counseling, and prayer.

Prenatal Testing

You will undergo a number of tests while pregnant. The most common are the AFP test, the ultrasound and, if you are above thirty-five or if your pregnancy is considered high risk, the amniocentesis or CVS test will also be performed.

The AFP Test

The AFP (alpha feto protein) test is done between the fifteenth and twentieth weeks of gestation. This tests for neural tube defects such as spina bifida and anencephaly. It is not a diagnostic test, but a screening test, meaning it does not diagnose a problem, but determines who is at increased risk and in need of further testing.

If your suspected dates of conception are at all off, an inaccurate abnormal result can occur, causing a great deal of anxiety. For this reason many providers offer routine ultrasound screening at this point in the pregnancy, which helps to confirm the dates of conception, making the AFP a more accurate test.

The Ultrasound

For the most part it has become routine for all women to have an ultrasound (also called a sonogram) between the sixteenth and eighteenth week. Through the use of sound waves this test creates a picture of the fetus and provides information about its development, such as age and rate of growth. It also confirms the date of conception and determines the overall health and viability of the fetus and placenta.

The Amniocentesis

If a woman is over thirty-five or presents specific high-risk health concerns, either an amniocentesis or a CVS sampling will also be done. By drawing a sample of the amniotic fluid from the amniotic sac, the amniocentesis test detects chromosomal problems, like Down's syndrome and other birth defects. It is not uncommon to experience uterine cramping and there is a less than 1 percent chance of miscarriage following this procedure. Like the ultrasound, the amniocentesis is administered at the sixteenth week of pregnancy.

CVS Sampling

A CVS (chorionic villus sampling) test examines the cells from the placenta to detect the same problems as an amniocentesis, but is done at around twelve weeks. The rate of miscarriage following it is slightly higher than that of the amniocentesis.

Genetic Testing

As prenatal care becomes more refined, genetic counseling becomes more widespread. Women who are at risk for birth defects or inherited conditions are referred to genetic counselors as early in their pregnancy as possible. These include women with a family history of inherited conditions or birth defects, those who are over thirty-five years of age, have had an abnormal ultrasound, have received abnormal results from screenings, or have experienced possible harmful exposures during pregnancy.

There are some carrier screenings that are ideally performed prior to becoming pregnant. These will detect if you are a carrier for a variety of diseases. If a woman tests positive for a genetic condition, her partner will then be screened. Some of the common ones that are tested for are:

* **Thalassemia**, a complex anemia occurring in Asian, Mediterranean, and African-American populations

* **Sickle cell diseases**, blood disorders occurring in African-American populations

* **Cystic fibrosis**, a lung and digestive system disease occurring in Caucasian populations

* **Tay-Sachs disease**, a disease of the brain and nerves occurring in Ashkenazi Jewish, French-Canadian, and Cajun populations

* **Canavan disease**, a disease of the brain and nerves occurring in Ashkenazi Jewish populations

A Difficult Choice

If only one parent is a carrier there is no risk of disease. When both parents are carriers for the same genetic disease there is a greater chance that the child will develop the disease. If this is the case, pregnancy termination will be an option. Some people who do not believe in pregnancy termination do not want genetic information in advance. Other people want information in advance, even if they plan to continue with the pregnancy. Other, very devout people believe that the fate of their baby is in God's hands but want information in advance in order to be prepared for what God is sending their way. After prenatal or genetic testing the pressure mounts for a woman and her partner to process the news and make a decision. It can be very trying on their relationship if they have differing beliefs and opinions about whether or not to terminate.

Even if this is not the case, the termination of a pregnancy is frightening and often traumatic. The procedure can take place in the obstetric unit of the hospital, close to where other women are laboring and giving birth, which can be terribly upsetting for a woman experiencing a loss. Some medical centers offer support groups for women (and their partners) who have experienced a pregnancy termination.

Conditions That Can't Be Determined Prenatally

There are other inheritable conditions, such as scoliosis and diabetes, that cannot be detected in advance. If you or your partner have such a disease it will be critical for you to know all the symptoms so that you can recognize them if they arise in your child.

Determining whether or not psychological and addiction disorders are part of a genetic legacy is a more complicated matter. There are a number of inquiries you might want to make so that you feel adequately informed. Is there a history of depression or any type of mental illness on either side of the family? Is there a history of addiction of any kind on either side of the family? These things will not necessarily manifest themselves, but it is good to know that there may be predispositions for them so that you can keep a watchful eye as your child matures.

High-Risk Pregnancies

Even before taking prenatal tests women with certain preexisting health conditions or atypical pregnancies are considered high risk from the outset. High-risk pregnancies are managed much more closely than routine ones. You will be considered high risk and likely managed by a high-risk specialist if you:

* Have a systemic disease, such as diabetes or a seizure disorder

* Have a drug abuse problem that impacts both you and your baby

* Are carrying multiple babies

* Learn that the baby is not growing normally

You will not be considered high risk, but your pregnancy will be monitored more closely if you:

* Have had previous miscarriages

* Develop gestational diabetes

* Have any type of preexisting health condition (high blood pressure, thyroid disease, cardiac condition)

* Are obese

* Have had a previous cesarean

* Are over thirty-five years of age

Like Mother Like Daughter?

One of the questions a childbirth educator hears the most is, "If my mother had an easy time conceiving, an uneventful pregnancy, or a quick labor with me, will I follow in her footsteps?" There have been no studies confirming whether or not this is the case. Although it does seem reasonable that if a mother and daughter have a similar menstrual pattern that a daughter's ability to conceive might mirror her mother's. Naturally, no two pregnancies or labors are exactly alike.

If My Pregnancy Goes Well, Won't Labor Be a Breeze?

There is no correlation between the personality of your pregnancy and the temperament of your labor. Ideally, if you are healthy and fit during your pregnancy, your labor will be relatively easy. But labor is unpredictable and a variety of issues can arise. As it is not necessarily the case that an easy pregnancy yields an easy labor, a difficult pregnancy does not necessarily result in labor that is hard, long, or fraught with complications.

Then and Now

Becoming pregnant in our current age of information and technology carries with it a different level of consciousness than in the past when there were fewer options and less awareness about women's health. Prior to the use of birth control in 1965, women were not able to effectively control conception. They generally had more children than they do now and it was expected that a woman would experience a miscarriage. There were no prenatal tests to predetermine the sex or health of the baby. If a woman were unable to conceive, whatever the cause, she would either remain childless or adopt a baby. Single motherhood was not a choice but a circumstance. Same-sex parents and families were unheard of. Options were far more limited, and woman's procreative health was something that was taken for granted.

So much has changed in a relatively short period of time and we can only expect more options (and, in certain circumstances, more confusion) as technology advances. And yet even with all the current knowledge and information there are no guarantees that you will become pregnant or give birth to a perfect baby. If you have challenges that feel insurmountable you might find yourself wishing you could walk in someone else's shoes. You may find yourself thinking, "This is all too big of a risk. I think I'll be just fine without a baby" or "Okay, so I'll say yes to the pregnancy decision, but only if I can know exactly what is going to happen." For some women things seem to fall into place with little effort. Others have to make challenging, sometimes painful choices. Each woman has her own individual path that leads her toward the pregnancy decision.

Making a Baby **Worksheet**

I know when I ovulate each month:

☐ Yes

☐ No

With each ovulation, I am most fertile ____ hours prior to ovulation.

At my age, the chances of becoming pregnant with each ovulation are ____ %.

The ways to tell if I am ovulating are:

The medical or genetic conditions I am concerned about are:

This is what I plan to do to improve my chances of becoming pregnant:

If I don't become pregnant right away it could be because:

If I don't become pregnant right away I will:

My attitude about becoming pregnant is:

Once I become pregnant, I will most likely have the following routine prenatal tests:

During pregnancy, I may be considered high risk if:

Given my ethnic background, I will need to have the following genetic screening test(s):

If I were to find out that my baby was at risk for a genetic disease I would:

3

Pregnancy after Thirty-five

The beauty of having a baby after thirty-five is that you approach the experience with wisdom that you didn't have when you were younger. You may be in better shape financially and reaping the benefits of years of personal growth in both your relationship with your partner and with yourself. You have learned and grown from a variety of life experiences. Your communication and conflict management skills have evolved with time and you may have more patience than you did when you were younger.

Bear in mind, though, that there are some unique concerns associated with this otherwise rosy picture. In addition to the decreased chances of conception, the physical changes of pregnancy and new motherhood might be more difficult to tolerate, particularly the early years of sleep deprivation. You may also have to face the reality, that, for better or for worse, you will have only one child. The good news is that most women over the age of thirty-five have problem-free pregnancies and healthy babies.

Carina, an athletic actress, became pregnant for the first time when she was thirty-five. Her partner already had a young son from a previous marriage. At sixteen weeks she was delighted to receive normal results from her amniocentesis. She gained thirty-two pounds and enjoyed swimming throughout her pregnancy. At thirty-nine weeks she gave birth to a healthy seven-pound boy. Her pregnancy and birth experience were not markedly different from a younger woman having her first baby. She felt fine both physically and emotionally. What Carina wasn't prepared for was the loss of sleep she would suffer during her son's first year of life. The postpartum period proved challenging for her, and she didn't return to feeling normal until well after her son's first birthday.

A generation ago, a woman over thirty-five having her first baby was over the hill. Traditionally, women began having children in their late teens and early twenties. Now, in the United States it is becoming more common for a woman to develop a career and wait until she is in the thirty to thirty-five bracket before she even begins considering pregnancy. In today's high-tech world, with our anything-is-possible mentality, women are having babies at forty-five. And we have all heard the amazing stories in the news about post-menopausal women becoming pregnant.

Issues Confronting the Thirty-five-and-Over Crowd

If you are over thirty-five and thinking of having a baby, your experience in becoming pregnant will differ in certain ways from that of your under thirty-five counterparts. Ovulation and fertilization are not as consistent in older women, and problems such as endometriosis and blocked fallopian tubes are more prevalent. The chances of becoming pregnant will not be as high as they were in your younger years.

Increased Risk Factors

Once you become pregnant your risk for certain complications increases. But this does not mean you are destined to experience problems. In fact, each day 1,000 U.S. women who are thirty-five and over give birth to healthy babies. Still, there is an increased risk of the following associated with pregnancy over thirty-five:

✳ Gestational (pregnancy induced) diabetes

✳ Hypertension (about 10 percent of women over thirty-five have elevated blood pressure)

✳ Placental abnormalities

✻ Miscarriage (by the time a woman is in her forties the risk is 50 percent, as opposed to 15 percent for a woman in her twenties)

✻ Low birth weight infant

✻ Stillbirth

Down's Syndrome

There is also a greater risk of chromosomal defects. Most notably, the risk of Down's syndrome increases with age. If you are almost or over forty, genetic counseling will help you assess the chances of giving birth to a baby with Down's syndrome and is strongly recommended. The odds of having a baby with Down's syndrome increase significantly if you are between thirty and forty-five.

Cesarean Births

The rate of cesarean births is twice as high for women in the thirty-five and older camp than for those under thirty-five. The reasons for this are unclear. Older women have their labors induced more frequently and have increased risk factors, such as hypertension and diabetes, that may contribute to the increased cesarean rate.

You and Your Genes

Women over thirty-five are advised to seek genetic counseling. This involves meeting with a doctor, nurse, or geneticist who will take a detailed family history and perhaps do a physical exam and a lab workup. The information gathered will help them gauge the risk of your having a baby with a birth defect. Along with the standard prenatal tests, such as the AFP and the ultrasound, there are others that women over thirty-five are offered (for more information on prenatal tests, see Chapter 2).

These include the amniocentesis and the CVS test, which provide critical information early in a pregnancy. When the results are not what they would have hoped for, women are faced with the choice of keeping or aborting the baby. If it has taken some time for a woman to conceive and the results of either the CVS or amniocentesis reveal a chromosomal abnormality, this choice can be very painful.

Darla had been pregnant three times since age thirty and had miscarried with each pregnancy. Finally, when she was thirty-six she became pregnant and, with a great deal of fear, made it to twelve weeks. Given Darla's concern, her doctor suggested she have CVS at this time, rather than waiting until sixteen weeks to do an amnio. When the results came back, she was told that her baby had Down's syndrome and was given the option of keeping the baby or having an abortion. She agonized for days. She had waited so long for this baby and after all the loss she'd experienced, didn't think she could bear having an abortion. She wasn't getting any younger and knew that from this point forward the odds of conceiving would only decrease. On the other hand, the thought of raising a child with such a serious problem worried her. She wondered if she'd have the emotional and physical wherewithal to cope, and feared her marriage might crumble under the strain of this challenge. The miscarriages had been difficult enough. She and her partner tried to weigh the positives and negatives so they could come to a rational, sensible decision. In the end Darla's choice emanated, not from her rational mind, but from a deep maternal sense within her. She decided to keep her baby.

The Most Important Thing

Good health prior to conception is of primary importance. If you have a prevailing health concern or condition, such as thyroid disease, diabetes, heart disease, or high blood pressure, you want to be sure that it is effectively managed before becoming pregnant. Once you set your sights on having a baby be sure to abstain from drugs, alcohol, and nicotine, and take vitamins with folic acid. Remember that fetal organs begin to form early on, at three to six weeks.

Fertility Counseling after Thirty-five

Because there is an overall decrease in the rate of conception and the ticking of the proverbial clock is a little louder, fertility counseling is typically more aggressive for women in this age group.

Rather than waiting a year before recommending a fertility workup, healthcare professionals might suggest intervention after just six months. Overall, women over thirty-five seek fertility evaluation twice as often as their under thirty-five counterparts.

Fertility Evaluation

A fertility evaluation consists of the following:

❋ Complete medical history

❋ Physical exam

❋ Blood test to check hormone levels

❋ Ovulatory function test

❋ Vaginal ultrasound to check the size, shape, and lining of the uterus and number of ovarian follicles

❋ HSG (hysterosalpingogram), an X ray of the uterus and fallopian tubes

❋ Sperm analysis of the father

Depending on the results, a laparoscopy, which is the insertion of a thin, lighted telescoping instrument into the abdomen to view the pelvic organs, might be indicated. This procedure would look for possible uterine fibroids or other problems in the uterus that might be preventing conception.

Fertility Treatment

The course of treatment will depend on the results of the fertility workup. Depending on age and the cause of infertility, it will be determined if you are a candidate for surgery or oral or injectable medication. Medications are often recommended to stimulate the ovaries to produce more eggs, increasing the potential for fertilization. How long this course of treatment lasts varies and at times it is given in combination with insemination.

Even before a more advanced course of fertility management is introduced, insemination treatment alone can cause unprecedented stress in a relationship. This often results in fights that seem as though they have been lifted from a not-so-funny sitcom.

> *Rebecca was driving through a Maine blizzard with a vial of her husband Marcel's fresh sperm in her pocket. When she reached the doctor's office where the insemination procedure was to take place, she was told that the sperm was no longer viable because it wasn't warm enough. She turned around and drove home in the blinding snow to retrieve yet another vial of sperm from her husband. When Marcel found out that she had driven with the sperm in her jacket pocket instead of between her legs, where it would have stayed warm, he became enraged and began screaming at her. After this incident, Rebecca began wondering, "Just how badly do I want a baby?"*

If a woman is not a good candidate for medication she might be considered for a high-tech intervention, such as in vitro fertilization (IVF) using her own or a donor's egg. IVF is also used when there are no fallopian tubes or they are blocked or damaged. The man's sperm and the woman's egg are fertilized in a laboratory dish and the resulting embryos are then transferred to the uterus. More than 100,000 babies have been born in the U.S. since 1981 as a result of IVF. But you should be aware that the pregnancy rate with IVF after age forty is low and most insurance plans do not cover this procedure.

Advanced infertility treatment is time-consuming and expensive, not to mention emotionally and physically draining. It can be very trying on a relationship; women who have difficulty conceiving often feel simultaneously angry, cheated, frustrated, and grief-stricken. Both women and their partners might experience feelings of self-blame, isolation, and helplessness. Psychological counseling or group support can be very helpful for a couple as they go through this process.

Some women go the full course of fertility treatment and still do not become pregnant. This can be disappointing, frustrating, and even heartbreaking. It almost always puts a major strain on a relationship. Some couples move forward and adopt a child. If the infertility is due to a problem with the sperm, sperm banks can be utilized. If surgery has left a woman without a uterus or she has a medical condition that will be aggravated by pregnancy, couples can hire a surrogate mother to carry a baby. If it is due to a problem with the egg, some couples seek out a donor egg.

Egg Donation

If test results indicate that there is no productive ovarian function, securing a donor egg could be the next step. There is a 55 percent pregnancy rate per cycle for women over forty who receive donor eggs. Following four cycles of egg donation, over 80 percent of women conceive. General criteria for egg donation are that you:

❋ Be over forty years of age

❋ Have high follicle stimulating hormone (FSH) levels at any age

❋ Have responded poorly to fertility medications in the past

❋ Have experienced age-related recurring miscarriage

❋ Have a normal uterus

Are There Other Options?

There are women who, after a lengthy period of fertility treatment with no results, abandon the Western medical model and seek other avenues. They go to healers of all varieties— homeopathic practitioners, acupuncturists, energy healers, spiritual healers, Chinese herbal specialists, and many different types of body workers. Though there is no scientific data supporting the efficacy of these alternative therapies, some women report that they have had luck with them.

Dora and her husband were Baptist missionaries who lived in both Taiwan and the United States. When she was thirty-four and their son, Matthew, was eight they decided to have another baby. She had become pregnant with Matthew within three months and figured her experience this time around would be similar. After a year of trying, Dora was unable to conceive. She agreed to fertility treatment and a year later was still not pregnant. When she returned to Taiwan the following year, a friend told her about a Chinese herbalist whose treatment had helped shrink her uterine fibroids. Dora had never been much into alternative medicine, but she was so disillusioned after trying to conceive for two years that she thought,

"I might as well check this out." The herbalist gave her a medley of herbs and after taking them for three months she became pregnant.

Stress after Thirty-five

When it comes to pregnancy there are certain stress points that are unique to the thirty-five and over age group. Because your lifestyle and identity are more defined you may experience many more doubts about jumping into such a big change. Certainly this state of ambivalence can characterize the decision-making process of a younger woman as well, but the crucial difference is that the younger woman knows that she can shelve the decision and then revisit it in a year or two. The ever-present ticking of the clock intensifies the level of tension for a woman and her partner.

> *After twelve years of being together, Lara, age thirty-nine, and her partner Paul began talking about the idea of becoming parents. Once discussion began, Lara vacillated daily. One day she would see herself all aglow pushing a stroller through the park; the next day she would have visions of herself trudging along in a walker at her child's high school graduation. She had spent the past ten years building a solid career as an architect and was ambivalent about letting go of the position she had worked so hard to achieve. On the other hand, she knew if she didn't bite the bullet and say yes now, that her chances of becoming a mother would rapidly diminish in the coming years. She would lie in bed at night wishing she had thought about this at age thirty. Paul had his share of ambivalence too, making it difficult for the two of them to reach a meeting of the minds.*

Then arises the question, "Is my relationship strong enough to survive pregnancy and parenthood?" If the pregnancy decision is fraught with difficulty, if just making the decision is straining the relationship, this will heighten the concern that it may not be able to withstand the pressures of parenting.

> *Thirty-four-year-old Whitney and her boyfriend, Josh, had been living together for five years when she began to feel the stirring desire to have a baby. When Whitney opened the discussion about becoming pregnant with Josh, who was*

thirty-six, he was adamantly against the idea. He didn't feel ready financially or emotionally. For the next six months, every time the topic of having a baby came up a heated argument ensued. They could not come to an agreement on this issue. Whitney had to come to the realization, that, though Josh had been her partner for over five years and she loved him, they were not going to have children together. Because she desperately wanted a baby, she decided she would have to let go of this relationship and try to find another man who felt ready. Their inability to find common ground on this issue was too big a hurdle to overcome as a couple.

Women in Whitney's situation, who want a baby sooner rather then later, have less time to spend negotiating with a partner who isn't ready for parenthood. Also, because many over thirty-fivers feel that they have only one chance at parenthood, they can develop an obsessive need to do everything right: to have the perfect pregnancy, labor, and birth, and to raise a flawless child. This can be stressful, particularly for an over thirty-five mother who is indeed having only one child. It also can put an inordinate amount of stress on the only child.

Of course, this is not always the case. Many women over thirty-five, with wisdom and experience on their side, are more relaxed and easygoing about pregnancy than they might have been when they were younger.

Will My Body Ever Be the Same?

For some over thirty-fivers, the overriding stress point is fear of losing their shape and not being able to regain or maintain it after childbirth. These women have had a longer time to develop eating and exercise habits that keep them at their optimal weight and there is a lot of fear associated with letting go of and redefining their regimen to meet the needs of pregnancy. It's not so easy to convince a woman who has been keeping her body in tip-top shape for years that pregnancy won't change things dramatically. The reality is that if you have long maintained a healthy weight and good overall fitness before pregnancy you will likely have an easy time maintaining a good weight throughout it and into the postpartum period. Unless, of course, you abandon your healthy eating habits in favor of a quart of ice cream a day!

The Sudden Loss of Control

As women mature they may have a more difficult time giving up control. They have been used to having things just so, in both their home and at work. Pregnancy is not something over which any of us has control. As you already have seen, conception might take some time, regardless of how healthy a lifestyle you maintain. You might experience severe nausea for most of your pregnancy, end up on bed rest for the last two months, or go into labor three weeks early. Going with the flow might not be so easy. It can also be a challenge for some older mothers to give up the personal time that they are so accustomed to having.

Because of all these issues, women over thirty-five may choose to have only one child, though this choice comes with mixed emotions. On the one hand this allows you to give your undivided attention to your child. On the other you may find yourself feeling guilty and selfish for not having more children.

Kumi, a dancer and choreographer, got married when she was thirty-six and had her first baby at thirty-eight. Her pregnancy was relatively easy, though labor was much more strenuous than she had imagined. By the time her daughter was a year old, Kumi was sure that she did not want any more children. Another child would result in a huge financial strain and would compromise her ability to pursue her artistic vision. She also liked the idea of being able to give her undivided attention to one child. Both her brother and sister had three children and the cousins spent a lot of time together, so she figured that her daughter, Gemma, would not be lonely. Although she believed her decision to have only one child a sound and reasonable one, Kumi still occasionally felt guilty and selfish for not having more children.

When the Past Affects the Present

Some women over thirty-five have had prior pregnancy experience. Some have had a child with an earlier partner or given a child up for adoption. Some have had abortions or lost a baby to miscarriage or stillbirth. Many of these women are with a new partner and beginning to look at life through new eyes. Often their concerns and feelings differ from those of a woman who is pregnant for the first time.

Maria had a nineteen-year-old daughter from a previous marriage. She became pregnant with her second child at age thirty-eight with her second husband Anthony. They lived in California while her daugher, Christina, was attending an East Coast college. When the baby was born, Christina, who had been supportive and loving throughout the pregnancy, became so infused with jealousy that she stopped speaking to her mother. Maria felt torn between her new family and her daughter and experienced a lot of guilt about loving her newborn. Christina's reaction made the transition to parenthood much more difficult for Maria and Anthony.

Arianna had given up her first child for adoption. Years later, at age thirty-six she became pregnant again. When she and her husband, Bud, met with their childbirth educator, Arianna, told the story of her earlier pregnancy. She was eighteen at the time and ill equipped to deal with the emotional turmoil the experience generated. When she and Bud made the decision to become pregnant it brought up a lot of emotions about the first baby, feeling that she had never allowed herself to experience. Her second pregnancy made her feel thankful for having another chance at motherhood, but it also aroused feelings of guilt and sorrow for the loss of her first child.

A Good Trade-off

Some women are relieved to finally let go of their careers, especially if they have become all-consuming. For them, the opportunity to love and nurture a baby is worth far more than the perks of their career status. For a woman accustomed to dealing with the rigors of the workforce, letting go of her career to be a full-time mom can be a very enticing proposition.

Of course, not all women are career minded and there are still some who don't work. For these women the changes of a baby take a different form. Women over thirty-five are typically more secure in their identity and becoming a mom does not feel as threatening as it might to a younger woman who is still trying to forge her identity.

Gladys had been working as a legal secretary since her early twenties. When she was thirty-seven she and her partner decided to have a baby. They agreed that she would work through her pregnancy and then stay home with the baby. She had been in the workforce for nearly twenty years and had always been a diligent worker who enjoyed the challenges and rewards of her career. She wanted to stay home with her baby but wondered how it would feel to let go of her work. Once Madeline was born, any doubt she had receded into the background. She loved being a mother and wanted nothing more than to be with her baby full-time. She had no interest in maintaining her career.

Fewer Raised Eyebrows

In today's world there remain cultures in which women have babies at a young age. In certain religious communities, for example, it would raise many eyebrows for a woman to wait until thirty-five to have her first baby. However, in many parts of the world an older mother does not turn heads in surprise. This means that over thirty-fivers can find the same support and companionship that younger mothers enjoy.

Undeniably, there are special concerns associated with having a baby later in life, but the majority of these pregnancies prove problem free. For most women over thirty-five the message is a resounding, "Go for it!"

Pregnancy after Thirty-five **Worksheet**

As a woman over thirty-five thinking about pregnancy, I feel more prepared than I was five years ago because:

Some of the complications I could possibly experience during pregnancy are:

Some of the stress points I might experience while pregnant are:

I feel prepared to handle this stress at this point in my life because:

4

A Healthy Lifestyle

Imagine that you are going to a prepregnancy spa for the next few months, or even years, until you become pregnant. See just how good you can be to yourself. The self-pampering can include a new exercise program, an improved diet, body work, massage, leisurely walks, gardening, meditation, and hot baths. The options are endless.

Believe it or not you can assimilate some of these self-nurturing techniques into your everyday life, and now is the time to do it. When you become pregnant, and certainly after giving birth, the focus of your energies will be mostly on your child, so use this time to secure habits that will promote health and well-being.

The formula for healthy living is:

❋ Eat properly.

❋ Exercise regularly.

❋ Overcome bad habits or addictions.

❋ Avoid risk factors in your environment.

❋ Keep your stress level to a minimum.

❋ Get a blood pressure check and if you've been told it's high, follow your doctor's orders for reducing it. This will minimize your chances of developing preeclampsia (a metabolic disorder that includes elevated blood pressure) in pregnancy.

You want to be in shape and at a good weight prior to becoming pregnant. Your doctor, nurse practitioner, or midwife will recommend that you gain between twenty-five and thirty-five pounds. Slimmer women often have to gain an extra five to ten pounds just to be at a good "fighting weight" for pregnancy, labor, and birth. Women carrying twins gain as much as forty-five pounds. This is a departure from times past when women were told that a weight gain of no more than fifteen pounds was normal.

Developing Healthy Eating Habits

Now is the ideal time to evaluate your diet and implement changes in it. The first step is to become aware of the types of food you eat. You may already be eating a healthy diet and in that case, this information will be a review. Because there are currently so many diet philosophies based on things like body type, particular health issues, moral beliefs, and cultural attitudes it is impossible to suggest a "one size fits all" diet. However, there are some general prescriptions for a healthy diet that can be addressed. It is recommended that you make diet changes three months to a year prior to conception.

Become a Label Checker

It can be an eye-opener to go to the grocery store, and rather than mechanically grab the products you are accustomed to buying, check their labels before putting them into your cart. If you aren't already a label checker, become one. You'll be surprised.

You may notice that some of your favorite foods are laden with sugar, salt, and fat. Snack bars, candy, and some breakfast cereals are packed with sugar; and excess sodium is found in some perennial American favorites, such as pizza, pickles, and chips. Foods like cheese, pastries, and nonlean red meat top the list of high-fat fare. Also, be aware that processed foods such as frozen dinners and sandwich meats, foods with dyes in them such as certain breakfast cereals and a variety of candy items, are notoriously high in sodium and nitrates. It is also best to avoid artificial sweeteners because they have no nutritional value.

Go for Organic

A general rule of thumb when altering your diet to prepare for pregnancy is: Eat fresh, organic food whenever possible. People are becoming increasingly aware of the value of eating organic produce, and more and more communities have open-air markets where you can buy fresh produce from organic farmers and/or an organic produce section in their regular grocery store. If organic is not available, be sure to rinse all fruits and vegetables to remove the chemicals from the skin.

No Time to Cook?

You may be thinking that you have no time for the additional amount of preparation that fresh foods require, but with creative planning you can fit this new activity into your life. It might work for you to spend a block of time on the weekend preparing food for the week. Some people cook in bursts and freeze for the future. Consider that once you are a parent you will want to spend time cooking and eating meals together as a family. So why not get started now?

End Your Relationship with Junk Food

Fast, deep fried foods like burgers and fries are full of fat, sugar, and sodium, which is of course why they are so seductively delicious. Unless you have an amazingly rapid metabolism, these foods are your enemies if you are trying to control your weight, not to mention your cholesterol levels. Sometimes it is hard to go cold turkey with a food that you have adored and is part of your regular diet. So try cutting back. Instead of three to four fast-food indulgences a week, try to have only two. Substitute with fresh, whole foods. You will probably find that you feel better and may give up the food altogether. Weight control is essential for you. Babies born to obese women are more at risk. If you are planning to lose weight, losing one to two pounds a week is a safe rate. Crash dieting can deplete the body's nutritional stores.

The Role of Protein

Protein is a valuable part of a daily diet for all women at whatever stage of life. If you are a person who does not gravitate toward protein, consider that once you are pregnant your need for it will increase. It is not uncommon for a woman who has been a committed vegetarian for years to have cravings for meat and become a meat eater while pregnant.

> *Since she was sixteen Holly had been a devout vegetarian with a fairly meager appetite. For both health and moral reasons, she had no intention of ever eating meat again. When she was twenty-five and in her first trimester she was nauseated more often than not, and tried to eat as simply as possible. Magically, as she progressed into her second trimester, the nausea lifted and her appetite came alive. No longer satisfied with a light salad or bowl of soup, she became a hearty meat and potatoes gal. Her partner barely recognized her, when after picking up dinner from the steakhouse, she came through the door and announced, "Hi, hon. We're having steak for dinner!"*

Your pregnant body will require a minimum of two servings of protein each day, which may be far more than you are currently consuming. Protein is necessary for the growth of the uterus and breasts, the growth of the placenta and baby, the development of muscles and the nervous system, and red blood cell formation. If you are a vegetarian, you will need to meet your protein needs with foods such as tofu and other soy products, beans and rice, and cheese and eggs.

Got Calcium?

All women, pregnant or not, benefit from getting 1000 to 1500 mg of calcium a day, and eating calcium-rich foods such as milk, yogurt, cottage cheese, cheese, and sesame seeds. It maintains strong bones, decreasing the overall risk of osteoporosis. Once pregnant, there is an increased need for calcium as your baby grows. Calcium is necessary for the growth of the uterus and breasts, the growth of the placenta and baby, formation of strong bones and teeth, increased blood volume, and the development of muscles and the nervous system. During pregnancy, a fetus grabs calcium from your system for bone development. If you are not taking in enough, it is you who will become calcium depleted, not the fetus. Women who are not big milk drinkers or who are lactose intolerant worry that they will not be able to ingest enough calcium while pregnant. Others experience severe leg cramps in pregnancy, which can be reversed by increasing calcium. If you happen to be like one of these women, you can take 2000 mg. a day as a supplement throughout your pregnancy in addition to eating other calcium-rich foods.

The Amount Counts

In addition to considering the quality of the food you eat, you want to consider the quantity per serving, as well as how often you eat. Some body conscious women have their own little tricks to control their weight. For example: Overeat on Monday, starve yourself on Tuesday; eat too much for breakfast, then eat minimally for the rest of the day; binge on sweets one evening and fast the next day. These sorts of irregular habits (certainly inadvisable at any time) are not recommended during pregnancy or prior to it. Regularly timed intake of food and liquid is very important to maintain optimal fetal growth and regulate maternal digestion and blood sugar. If you begin eating regular, moderately sized meals now, by the time you become pregnant it will be second nature.

Changes in Appetite

Appetite itself varies from woman to woman. For many women, pregnancy is a time of increased, perhaps even voracious appetite and appreciation of food. It is not unusual for a woman to be hungry every two hours and require frequent healthy snacks to keep her blood sugar levels regulated. Some women brag about eating their husbands under the table for the first time. It can really be a kick for a woman who has eaten like a bird for most of her life to have such a hearty appetite. Other women have little interest in food and need to force themselves to eat the minimum amount necessary to maintain weight gain.

Hang Out at the Water Cooler

Because a woman's body fluid increases by 40 percent during pregnancy, your daily liquid intake becomes essential. Most women do not take in an adequate amount of fluid before becoming pregnant. Why not increase your fluid intake now in preparation for being pregnant? Try drinking six to eight glasses of water a day, if you aren't already in the habit. Of course you then have to make frequent visits to the rest room. If a pregnant woman does not drink enough throughout the day she may have problems.

Cynthia, who drove ten-hour shifts as a truck driver, would go without fluids the entire day and drink in the evening when she got home. At the end of her first trimester she experienced severe abdominal pain and went to the emergency room, fearing she was in labor. It turned out that she was severely constipated due to lack of fluid.

Cravings

We hear a lot about the cravings that women develop while pregnant, such as the peculiar ritual of eating pickles and ice cream together. There are those who claim that a woman craves foods that offer nutrients she is lacking in her diet. Others believe that women gravitate toward comfort food, such as salty or sweet snacks. Sometimes women suddenly fall in love with a food they have never liked before, such as artichokes, chopped liver, or beets. Cravings can also be related to both smell and color.

Andrea, during her second trimester, would beg her husband to drive thirty minutes to a specific Thai restaurant in North Hollywood that had a particular kind of egg roll. Once the order was handed to her, she would smell it and then give it to her husband to eat. And this happened more than once!

Don't Forget Your Vitamins

You can also begin prenatal vitamins, which have added folic acid, in advance. There are various opinions regarding which type of prenatal vitamins are the best. Your provider will prescribe one that you can pick up at a pharmacy. Be aware that vitamins, particularly the iron in them, might upset your stomach, especially in the first trimester. But it is not a good idea to eliminate the iron because without it there is a higher risk of anemia. It might be helpful to take them at night before bed or with food so they digest more easily. Some people prefer to take individual vitamins rather than an all-in-one prenatal supplement. If you choose your own vitamins, make sure that you first receive professional guidance regarding the kind and amounts to take. Oversupplementation during pregnancy can be harmful to the health of the growing fetus.

Food Rich in Folic Acid

Folic acid is crucial in decreasing the risk of brain and spinal cord (neural tube) defects. The March of Dimes reports that folic acid decreases the risk of neural tube defects by 50 to 70 percent. It is recommended, that, beginning a year in advance and during your pregnancy, you enrich your diet with 400 micrograms of folic acid daily. Foods that are high in folic acid are broccoli, kale, spinach, citrus fruits, nuts, legumes, liver, whole grains, and fortified breads and cereals.

How Much Weight Will I Gain?

Weight gain in pregnancy is a worrisome topic for many women. The fear of fat can even discourage some women from becoming pregnant and cause others to eat an inadequate diet during pregnancy. Some people (sometimes including the pregnant woman herself) refer to a pregnant woman as "fat," which perpetuates a negative self-image. As previously mentioned, a healthy pregnant woman is expected to gain twenty-five to thirty-five pounds. The typical breakdown of this weight gain is as follows:

Four to six pounds	Maternal stores (fat, protein, and other nutrients)
Two to three pounds	Increased fluid
Three to four pounds	Increased blood
One to two pounds	Breast growth
Two pounds	Uterus
Six to eight pounds	Baby
Two pounds	Amniotic fluid
One to two pounds	Placenta

Women who are significantly overweight are expected to gain only about fifteen pounds. When a woman gains substantially more weight than is appropriate, either due to poor eating habits, severe edema (swelling), or some other medical condition, then there may be some increased risk for problems.

This is why one of the most critical things you can do for yourself and your baby is to begin your pregnancy at a healthy, stable weight. Obesity in pregnancy can negatively impact blood glucose levels and blood pressure.

Conversely, there are women who have trouble gaining weight during pregnancy, which can also be problematic. These women often have to force-feed themselves a high-calorie diet at regular intervals in order to maintain even a minimal weight gain. If the baby is not growing properly, they are put on bed rest for the third trimester. The struggle to maintain a healthy weight for an underweight woman can feel just as difficult, and create as much anxiety, as the struggle that an overweight woman experiences.

If, during pregnancy, concerns regarding nutrition and weight gain arise, consultation with a nutritionist will be recommended. He or she can help you design a manageable diet that will provide all the nutrients your growing baby needs.

Exercise

Once you become pregnant, it is not recommended that you begin a new, challenging exercise routine. It is fine, however, to begin low-stress activities such as yoga or walking, which promote strength and endurance while relieving stress. Badminton and croquet are also low stress. The American College of Obstetrics and Gynecology once recommended limits on exercise duration and heart rate. The current recommendation is that women with uncomplicated pregnancies can enjoy exercise throughout the nine months. A general rule of thumb is if you become too breathless to talk while exercising, your heart rate is too high. Wear comfortable, supportive clothing (support bra and exercise shoes), do not become overheated, and stay hydrated while exercising. You always want to allow for warm-up and cool down time at each exercise session. Before beginning any prenatal routine, check with your provider to make sure you have no health restrictions. Many programs require a letter of consent from your health care provider.

Today is a great day to begin exercising if you have not yet done so. Pick something that is safe and that you enjoy doing frequently. Regular exercise promotes bone and muscle growth, increases muscle tone, strength, endurance, and energy. It also improves mood and posture, aids digestion, and helps you sleep well.

If you enjoy being outdoors, brisk walking and some light free weights might be just the ticket. Some people are crazy about running steps, playing tennis, or using the cardio equipment at the gym. Find the program that best suits your temperament, your schedule, the weather in your part of the country, and your finances. Mix and match different forms and become a cross trainer.

During pregnancy exercise relieves constipation, swelling, and bloating; decreases back pain; and gives you extra strength and endurance for coping with labor. Certain sports such as skiing, horseback riding, and water skiing are not recommended. Scuba diving is a sport that is both difficult and contraindicated because it puts the fetus at risk for an air embolism.

When pregnant you want a form of exercise that will increase flexibility, strength, and endurance. If you adopt a fairly strenuous program prior to pregnancy, it will have to be modified once you are pregnant. For example, running steps, heavy weight lifting, skiing, and intense aerobic activity are contraindicated. Your joints will become looser due to the hormone relaxin, which relaxes ligaments, making them more susceptible to injury. Intense heart-elevating exercise will increase blood and oxygen flow to the muscles being worked and away from the uterus. Because your center of gravity shifts due to extra weight, more stress is placed on joints and muscles in the pelvis and lower back.

In pregnancy, avoid movements that are jarring or jerky and avoid overstretching. Your loose ligaments may allow your body more range of motion, which could result in injury. Do not exercise to the point of exhaustion, and if you feel pain, light-headed, or out of breath, stop immediately. In general women tend to prefer swimming, walking, stationary biking, prenatal exercise or prenatal yoga classes. Dancing is also great exercise and a wonderful form of self-expression.

People often have interesting advice about what you should and shouldn't do while pregnant. It is always a good idea to check your source.

During Lola's first pregnancy she had been told by her Aunt Sonia that dancing would cause the umbilical cord to wrap around the baby's neck. Brazilian dance, her obsession, kept her body in shape and her spirits high. It had been very diffi-cult for her to stop. In her sixth month she joined a prenatal exercise class at the YWCA, figuring it would be sedate enough to avoid any complications. One evening the teacher put on some Latin music and all the women danced. She told her instructor what her aunt had said about dancing and dis-covered that it was an old wives' tale. Think of all that great dancing she missed!

Walking and swimming are very easy on the joints and muscles. When swimming, you don't sweat and feel weightless, which is refreshing. You may find that you have more stamina for swimming laps than doing repetitions in an exercise class. Swimming is very helpful for increasing stamina and breath con-trol. If you are pregnant in the summer, there's not much that beats being in cool water. Here's a summer tip for pregnant women: Go to the beach and dig a hole in the wet sand. Lie on your stomach in the hole and relax. Enjoy the feeling of resting on your stomach again.

In prenatal exercise classes you will do a combination of stretching and strengthening exercises and low-impact aerobics, often set to upbeat music. You will have the chance to get to know other pregnant women and talk about your discomforts and concerns. Often centers that offer prenatal classes also have postnatal classes, giving you the opportunity to be part of a com-munity of women.

The Yoga Connection

Adopting a yoga practice can be beneficial for women before becoming pregnant. Not only does yoga increase your physical strength and balance, but it gives you stress reduction tools that can help you cope with your own personal prepregnant stress points.

Yoga consists of a variety of *asanas* or poses that are held as you breathe. The breathing contributes to a sense of inner balance and calm that is ideal preparation for labor. Unlike other forms of exercise, yoga addresses both body and spirit. You will learn poses like pelvic tilt, downward facing dog, tree, triangle, and squats. It is to be expected that the balance poses may become more challenging as pregnancy progresses. As the uterus grows larger, your center of gravity will change, just as it did in puberty. A number of fitness centers offer pre- and postnatal yoga classes. This gives you the opportunity to share concerns with other mothers-to-be and new moms, while forming a new social circle. In this setting pregnant women benefit from hearing other women's birth stories. Personal "before and after" involvement with other women can really decrease the fear of the unknown that preys upon most pregnant women.

Squatting

The squatting position is frequently practiced in yoga classes. It aids digestion, opens the pelvis, and takes strain off the lower back. Women often like to practice daily squatting in preparation for labor. This can be done with the support of a chair, in a corner with your back to the wall, with a partner's support, or in the middle of the room with no support if you are strong enough. Some women are natural squatters; others find it awkward or difficult. If a woman has hemorrhoids or a tendency toward getting them, she should have support under her buttocks while squatting. If a full squat is not comfortable, a half squat, done in a standing position, is fine. If you have bad knees, avoid squatting altogether.

There is a video made in Brazil entitled *Birth in the Squatting Position*, which shows a stunning series of women squatting for birth. Squatting is encouraged for the following reasons:

- It increases pelvic capacity by one to two cm. Any extra room you can create for the baby is of great benefit.
- You have gravity in your favor as you push to give birth, which aids in the descent of the baby.
- It helps the baby line up with the angle of the pelvis because the pelvis is well tilted when squatting.

Not all women are comfortable or strong enough for this. There are other positions a woman can assume for birth that will increase pelvic capacity.

Kegels

Ever heard of a kegel exercise? The pelvic floor muscles or perineum are a hammock of muscles surrounding the vagina and the rectum that support internal organs, such as the bladder and the uterus. These muscles are scarcely mentioned until a woman becomes pregnant. Then we start telling her to do one hundred kegel or pelvic floor exercises per day. By practicing kegels you train yourself to become conscious of this area, so that when you are pushing you can differentiate between a relaxed and tense perineum. These muscles undergo tremendous stress during childbirth, so keeping them toned will minimize the chance of a prolapsed bladder or uterus later in life. A Kegel is simply the contracting and releasing of the pelvic floor muscles. Once you are in your childbearing years it is recommended that you do a hundred of these a day. Women find inventive ways to fit kegels into their daily routine.

Toby does her kegels to the tick of her bedside clock each night.

Martha does five to ten during each commercial break while watching television.

Alicia prefers to practice kegels while having sex. Her child-birth educator taught her "elevator" kegels, which are done by contracting the vaginal muscles little by little like an elevator ascending.

If you drive, you can squeeze in five to ten kegels per red light. It is not too early to start them now to be ahead of the learning curve. It is recommended that you do these even after the childbearing years into mid- and later life to keep the pelvic floor muscles in good shape. This is helpful if you have problems with incontinence after menopause.

Strengthening Your Lower Back

Because your abdominal muscles lose much of their tone during pregnancy, you end up relying on your back to do some of the work your abs once did (and will do again!). It is advantageous to go into a pregnancy with a strong lower back. Strengthening exercises, such as pelvic tilts, are recommended. They can be done on hands and knees, standing, or on the back, though this position is not recommended for sustained periods of time in pregnancy, especially after twenty weeks, because the weight of the uterus presses on the main artery (vena cava), cutting off oxygen to the baby. Certain yoga postures and weight machines at the gym strengthen lower back muscles. You can also do minisit-ups during pregnancy. When done safely in a modified form, these minimize stress on the lengthwise abdominal muscles, which can separate in pregnancy.

The Mechanics of Movement

As the baby grows and your body changes, you will probably feel challenged by the body mechanics of simple tasks. No longer able to see your toes, you might wonder, "How exactly do I pick up a bag of groceries or tie my shoe?" Using the large muscle groups, e.g., the arms and the legs for strength whenever possible in order to relieve stress on both the back and abdominal muscles is recommended. For example, the suggestion for picking up and carrying grocery bags is: Squat, bring the bag close to your chest, and use the strength of the legs to get back up. When lying down, lie first on the side, then gently move onto the back; when getting up, move back onto the side, using the strength of the arms to push up to a seated position. It is too much stress on the abdominal wall muscles to lie directly on or push directly up from being on the back.

Doing gentle weight lifting and other upper body strengthening exercise prior to pregnancy will be of great benefit in moving through pregnancy and nursing, not to mention carrying both the baby and all the paraphernalia that becomes part of your life. Once pregnant, it is important to be mindful of body mechanics and stay balanced while stair climbing, chair sitting, shoe tying, and putting on your panty hose. For toenail painting it is best to ask for help from a partner, pal, or pedicurist!

A Good Time to Break Bad Habits

Given the choice, it is not in your best interest or that of your baby to wait until you are pregnant to overcome an addiction. If you start cleaning up your life now in regards to drug, alcohol, nicotine, and caffeine consumption, your body will be that much stronger and healthier when you become pregnant. Also, there will be less risk that your baby's health will be impacted by a harmful substance that you are choosing to ingest.

It is fascinating just how many lifestyle changes a woman will make for the sake of her baby, but not for herself. Women stop smoking and drinking, give up coffee, overcome drug addictions, change their diets dramatically, begin exercising, and learn to reduce stress in order to create optimal fetal health. Some of these changes are obviously easier to make than others. Sometimes bad habits, such as lack of exercise or eating too much candy, are hard to break. While these are not ideal, childbirth educators and health care providers do not worry that they will cause severe harm to a fetus. The threat associated with substance abuse, whether it is engaged in chronically or as part of a bingeing pattern, is far more dangerous when a woman is pregnant. Even rare use of certain substances, such as cocaine, can cause vasoconstriction and morbidity. If you use a substance frequently and are not able to quit, this is a good indication that it is time to ask for help. Among available resources are your doctor, the chemical dependency program offered by your health insurance plan, and twelve-step programs in your community. You can also find local referrals and services by calling local information. It is imperative for you to abstain from substances as you are trying to conceive because they can severely harm a developing fetus in the first weeks of pregnancy.

It is also important to remember that all substances cross the placenta and enter the baby's bloodstream. Three and a half weeks gestation is the most vulnerable period for a developing fetus, though you want to abstain throughout pregnancy because certain substances are more risky later. Risks include miscarriage, low birth weight, SIDS, mental retardation, physical defects, and learning disabilities. There is never an amount you can ingest that will be safe for your developing baby.

Alcohol

Alcohol, commonly believed to be the most innocuous of substances, ingested during pregnancy has very serious repercussions for both you and your baby. You will be at greater risk for both miscarriage and preterm labor. Your baby will be at risk for

FAS (fetal alcohol syndrome), which causes permanent physical defects and mental retardation. Providers, for the most part, recommend complete abstinence during pregnancy, though some say a celebratory sip of wine, champagne, or beer is okay. You can also put your baby at risk by binge drinking—consuming five or more alcoholic drinks on one occasion. A fetus exposed to a high blood alcohol concentration even once is at greater risk for developing problems with behavior and brain function. Even if the baby appears healthy at birth, the long-term consequences of alcohol use are not known.

> *Amy and her boyfriend Roger were very edgy the last evening of their childbirth preparation class. When the class ended, they stayed late to talk with the instructor. Amy told her that during her first trimester, before discovering she was pregnant, she had been drinking a lot and often with friends. She had been unable to discuss this with her doctor, and throughout the pregnancy had suffered a great deal of anxiety because of it. Once she opened up and told her instructor, she and Roger both began to cry, they were so worried about their baby. The instructor did her best to allay their fears, not knowing herself what affect Amy's alcohol consumption might have had on the developing fetus. When they left they felt relieved that they had finally talked to someone.*

Nicotine

Nicotine, which some people forget is a drug, has a number of side effects when used during pregnancy, including reduced oxygen flow to the fetus and a doubled risk of low birth weight. Twenty to 41 percent of women smokers spontaneously quit when they learn they are pregnant. Approximately 70 percent of these women will lapse back into smoking within a year of giving birth. Pregnant smokers have a 25 percent greater risk of fetal or infant death with their first baby if they smoke less than a pack a day, and a 50 percent greater risk if they smoke more than a pack a day.

A child of a mother who smoked during pregnancy is at greater risk for respiratory problems, delayed growth, and poor school performance. Current studies are also finding increased rates of ADHD (attention deficit/hyperactivity disorder) and criminal behavior in boys of mothers who smoked during pregnancy. Smoking cessation programs are available through certain health plans and community health organizations. As with all substances, you want to quit prior to becoming pregnant, although quitting once you become pregnant is still better than not quitting at all.

> *Suzanne attended a smoking cessation class during her fourth month of pregnancy. She had quit for the first two months when her nausea was so terrible she couldn't tolerate smoking. Once the nausea subsided, she found herself once again craving cigarettes at certain times throughout the day. Knowing how bad it was for her baby, she tried to overcome these urges on her own, but wasn't successful. Her nurse practitioner referred her to a special prenatal smoking cessation program. The class provided her with information, tools, and support— the three things she needed to overcome her addiction. She felt certain that she would be able to give up cigarettes for the duration of the pregnancy, and hoped that once the baby was born her cravings would remain under control.*

Secondhand smoke is also of serious concern during pregnancy. If there is a smoker in your house, or you have visitors who smoke when they are with you, now is a good time to establish a no smoking rule in your home.

Caffeine

Caffeine is another substance that can negatively impact conception and the fetus. More than three cups a day of caffeine containing beverages may have an effect on fertility. During pregnancy, it speeds up the mother's metabolism, which in turn speeds up the baby's. Though coffee is the substance that first comes to mind when you mention caffeine, tea, chocolate, soda pop, cocoa, diet pills, No Doz, and certain pain relievers (Anacin, Excedrin) all have significant amounts of caffeine. Some providers encourage removing caffeine completely from the diet; most set a limit at two cups of coffee a day or the equivalent. The smell of coffee is typically offensive in the first trimester, at which point some women quit coffee altogether. Others switch to decaf, though this is most often chemically processed and still has a small percentage of caffeine.

Other Drugs

Drugs of any kind—over the counter, prescription, or recreational—are all off-limits during pregnancy, unless prescribed specifically by your physician. If you are involved with drugs now and planning a pregnancy, be aware that they can cause amennorhea (lack of menstruation), and without ovulation conception is impossible. Everything you ingest during pregnancy crosses the placenta, which means that any substance that alters your metabolism affects the baby.

The current use of psychotropic drugs gives rise to questions about the safety of mood-altering drugs during pregnancy. These issues must be discussed with both your physician and therapist.

Finding Support

If you have a substance abuse problem and are considering pregnancy, now is the time to make changes in your life. Many medical centers offer programs that provide you with skills to help change unhealthy behaviors through their health education centers, and numerous twelve-step programs are readily available. A regular exercise routine and an ongoing spiritual practice are both avenues that help many people as they struggle with these issues. In conjunction with a rehabilitation program or therapy, you might explore any of the following: talk therapy, support groups, meditation, chanting, yoga, tai chi, prayer, or journaling. If during your pregnancy you continue to use any type of substance you must let your provider know so that you can get appropriate counseling and medical care.

Environmental Toxins

In addition to those toxins that are ingested, there are external ones that can threaten the health of both the pregnant woman and the fetus. Avoid breathing in fumes of household cleaning products. Ideally, someone else should take over the chores that require these products. But if this is not an option, make sure you are in a room with an open window when using them. If you have the inside of your house or the baby's room painted, stay out of the house while it is being done, and when you return make sure the house is well ventilated. Stay away from paint thinner. Pesticides used in concentrated doses, either in the yard or to repel household insects such as fleas, should be avoided. Mercury exposure is also very dangerous. Toxoplasmosis, a disease transmitted through cat feces, is another danger for pregnant women. If you have a cat, someone else in the house will need to cover litter box duty. Substances in the home such as lead paint and asbestos can be poisonous to a child.

Changing Your Lifestyle and Sticking to It

There is a lot to digest when thinking about making lifestyle changes prior to becoming pregnant. It might feel like too much to take on and you may think, "I will never be able to climb these mountains. I can't possibly change my eating and exercise practices in order to prepare for pregnancy, not to mention my coffee habit. I might as well give up on my dream of being a mother." Or you might find yourself thinking, "None of these things I do are so bad. My mother smoked cigarettes and drank coffee when she was pregnant with me and I'm fine." Conversely, your response to this information may be, "I really do want a baby, and I feel ready to make any lifestyle changes that will help me live a healthier life and create a safer environment for my child."

As you consider the lifestyle changes you would like to make, remember you don't need to become a brand new person overnight. In fact, if you do pressure yourself to change your diet, exercise, and overall health habits all at once, it more than likely will not last. Take time to think about your lifestyle and slowly, mindfully alter your habits. If you feel unable to alter certain habits (for example, you may have an ideal goal of giving up coffee, but find it difficult to do so), modify them. If you have a substance abuse problem, address this issue before anything else. Quitting is the most critical lifestyle change you can make for the sake of your baby. Make these adjustments with compassion for yourself and consideration for your long-term health and well-being. You and your baby-to-be deserve it.

A Healthy Lifestyle **Worksheet**

In order to improve my health before becoming pregnant:

☐ There is nothing about my lifestyle I need to alter.

☐ There are several modifications I would like to make.

☐ There are some significant changes I would like to make.

☐ There are some major changes I need to make.

In order to make these changes:

☐ I don't need any help.

☐ I need help.

I plan to get help by:

☐ Seeing a nutritionist or other professional who can help me alter my diet

☐ Joining a weight management organization

☐ Joining a gym or health club

☐ Joining a yoga class

☐ Using exercise or yoga videotapes at home

☐ Starting my own exercise program, e.g., walking with friends

When considering the lifestyle changes I want to make to prepare for pregnancy, the ones that feel the most challenging to me are:

In order to maximize my health to prepare for pregnancy I will make the following changes in my diet:

In order to maximize my health to prepare for pregnancy I will make the following changes in my exercise habits:

I am currently doing the following for exercise:

I exercise ____ times a week for ____ minutes.

The cardiovascular component to my workout is:

In order to maximize my health to prepare for pregnancy I will make the following changes in my intake of harmful substances:

In order to help me overcome any substance abuse problems, I will:

- ☐ Seek the counsel and support of a twelve-step program.
- ☐ Consult a therapist who can help me deal with my substance abuse.
- ☐ Investigate rehabilitation programs offered through my insurance plan.
- ☐ Consult community-based organizations for referrals to various programs.

5

Get Practical before Pregnant

When it comes to health care, birth choices, and work-related issues, women sometimes make the unfortunate mistake of not researching their options in advance. As a result, they can wind up in situations that are not best suited to their needs. There is no better time than the prepregnancy stage to begin educating yourself on the practical matters that will determine how your pregnancy is handled. As you know, your needs will change once you become pregnant. Understanding your options is the first step to ensuring that those needs are fulfilled to your satisfaction. So use this time to gather information. Start thinking about who you want for your health care provider; whether you want to deliver in a hospital, birth center, or at home; what hospital you want to use; what you need from an insurance plan; and what kind of work schedule you need. It makes all the difference when these matters are settled beforehand.

What You Need to Know about Your Health Insurance

If your insurance is provided via your or your partner's employment, it is often the case that you do not have a say in which plan is assigned to you. Regardless, familiarize yourself with the details of your insurance plan, so you are well versed in what it offers. Some of the questions to keep in mind when reviewing your insurance are:

❀ What type of medical groups are covered?

❀ How many nights in the hospital are covered?

❀ Are private rooms covered?

❀ Do you have DME (durable medical equipment) coverage?

❀ Can you use a midwife if you choose to do so?

❀ Does it cover a lactation consultant?

❀ What will your total out-of-pocket expenses be for prenatal care, lab work, and inpatient stay?

Medical Groups

Depending on the type of coverage you have, you may or may not be able to choose a provider who will see you all the way through your prenatal care to the birth of your baby. This can depend not only on your insurance coverage, but also on whether you live in a rural or urban area. In small towns it is still possible to find a physician who will be the sole provider on call during your pregnancy and birth. If you live in a more cosmopolitan area and are able to choose your provider, you will find that most ob/gyn practices consist of a group of four or more providers. You will often rotate among them throughout your pregnancy, so that by your ninth month you will have met the entire group. In addition to M.D.s your provider group may include a nurse practitioner, a midwife, or a resident. Nurse practitioners are not licensed to do deliveries. Generally, the doctor who helps you during the birth will be the one in the practice who is on call. You may belong to an HMO where you have a consistent provider during the pregnancy, but give birth with whoever is on call in the hospital.

If you give birth in a teaching hospital, this physician may be a resident who has finished his or her medical training and is pursuing a specialty in ob/gyn. Because they are recently out of medical school residents come equipped with the most current medical training and knowledge. Still, if you want a closer bond with the care giver who presides over the delivery it can feel disconcerting to have an unfamiliar face in the room.

When Christina went into labor in the middle of the night, the doctor in her practice with whom she felt most comfortable was on call, so she felt reassured that she would get top-notch care while in labor. By the following morning her labor had not progressed much and the doctor's shift was ending. One of the other partners whom she wasn't terribly fond of was now on call. Christina's labor continued through the day and into the next night. By the time she began pushing, the doctor on call was someone she had never met and who was filling in for the third doctor in the practice. She was less than pleased that the doctor delivering her baby was a stranger. Luckily, this physician was very compassionate and helped make Christina's birth a joyous experience.

Julie went into her labor knowing that she might be cared for by an unfamiliar doctor. However, when it came down to the final push, she wanted to at least be introduced to this person before her baby was born. She had been pushing in a semirecline position with the nurse in attendance for about fifteen minutes, when a male doctor she had never laid eyes upon came into the room in the middle of a contraction. He sat facing her perineum and began giving her pushing advice. When the contraction ended, she lifted her head, held out her right hand and said, "Excuse me, but I would appreciate it if you would introduce yourself first before taking a front row seat."

Midwives

You may also want to investigate having a midwife as your primary care provider. There are two types of midwives. One is a certified nurse midwife (CNM) and the other a lay midwife. CNMs train for three years in a program that is geared toward hospital birth. Not all hospitals employ CNMs. Those that do include certain Kaiser medical centers and some community hospitals. Women who prefer a midwife during labor usually feel that she will spend more time, be more compassionate, and less interventionist than a doctor.

Lay midwives specialize in home birth. When interviewing a lay midwife you want to find out about her experience, education, and how she handles emergencies. Get references and ask about her backup physician. A competent and accessible backup team is imperative if you are leaning toward home birth. The doctors in your community may vary in their attitudes toward lay midwives.

When Eva was pregnant with her first child, she began researching the possibility of having a home birth. The midwife in her small town came highly recommended, so she scheduled an interview with her. During the interview she discovered that the doctors in her community were not supportive of home birth and none of them were willing to provide backup medical care. In the case of an emergency, Eva would be rushed to a medical center that was a forty-minute drive from her home. This was not an arrangement that she felt comfortable with, so Eva opted for an ob/gyn in her community who had a noninterventionist orientation.

Dena, a nurse, wanted a personal connection with the provider who facilitated her labor, instead of what she called the "invasion mentality" of the hospital. Ideally, she envisioned delivering in a birth center, so that her experience would be less medically oriented. Unfortunately, in her California town no such center was available, so she secured the services of a home birth midwife recommended by a friend. At their first meeting she felt an instant connection. For the first twenty weeks of pregnancy she also received care from her HMO, which included an ultrasound at sixteen weeks, but no AFP test or amniocentesis. The midwife used only her ear rather than a listening device to hear the baby's heartbeat and taught Dena's husband to do the same. She did no vaginal checks and had Dena take responsibility for her own care as much as possible. Prenatal care was offered every Friday from two to five in a group format. Because it is impossible for a lay midwife in the state of California to carry malpractice insurance, Dena and her husband signed a contract waiving their rights to sue. The fee was $3,000, which included all prenatal care, lab work, the birth, and postpartum follow-up care. Dena had her baby at home in a warm birthing pool. The midwife stayed with her for ten hours after the birth.

Start Researching Providers

Whether you think you want to use a midwife or an M.D., start researching providers in your community now, so that when it comes time to make a final choice you will be well informed. Get references and speak with women who have used the provider you are considering. This will help you gain some insight into their practice and philosophy. Certainly one of the tricky points of doing a lot of advance legwork these days is that jobs, and subsequently living situations, and health insurance coverage change like the wind. Even so, if you do extensive research in your community and end up not living there when you get pregnant, you will know what questions to ask and will have a better idea of what you want. It is also possible that you will find the care provider of your dreams and he or she will move by the time you become pregnant. Such is life in the modern world!

Choosing a Health Care Provider

What exactly is it you are looking for when choosing a care provider? It is customary in most communities for women to interview several potential providers before making a choice. Check in advance to make sure that there will not be a charge for the interview. Here are some of the questions you want to consider:

* Is the office in a convenient location?

* Is the office close to your home or work?

* Is there convenient parking available?

* Is the hospital that the provider is affiliated with close to your home?

* If there is a hospital you prefer, does the provider have privileges there?

* How is his or her bedside manner?

This last question should not be underestimated. When a doctor refers you to another doctor it is based on clinical expertise and reputation. This does not mean that this doctor has a bedside manner that will work for you. The provider who ushers you through your pregnancy becomes a very important person in your life. Make sure you feel comfortable asking questions and that your questions are answered to your satisfaction. It is important to feel safe and at home with this person.

How Is the Office Staff?

Remember that you will be dealing with a team of people, not just your physician. So ask yourself these questions about the staff at your provider's office.

❋ Are the people who answer the phones friendly?

❋ Do they keep you on hold for decades?

❋ Are they patient with you as they schedule your appointments?

❋ Do they return your phone calls? How quickly?

❋ Do they respond appropriately to your special needs or requests?

❋ Are the medical personnel in the office compassionate and friendly?

❋ Do they make eye contact with you when you come in?

❋ Do you feel comfortable with them?

What Is the Provider's Philosophy?

Think about the personal beliefs that are the most important to you and find a care provider who shares your values. For example, if you plan to breast-feed for at least a year, or to have a family bed, find someone who will support you in those choices.

How Available Is He or She in an Emergency?

If you were to have a medical emergency during your pregnancy and are with a medical group, it is most likely that the provider who is on call will meet you in the hospital emergency room. Find out what the on call system is in the group you choose. What if you have an emergency in the middle of the night? You want to be comfortable enough with your provider or provider group to call if you need medical advice or help at any hour of the night or day.

What Are His or Her Intervention Statistics?

Women often feel awkward about asking a doctor to reveal his or her intervention statistics. However, before selecting a provider, it is important that you be informed about his or her record. What is the provider's cesarean rate? According to the World Health Organization, the overall rate should not be over 10 to 15 percent, though most providers and hospitals have a rate that is between 20 and 25 percent. Rates for episiotomy (a cut done between the vagina and the rectum to allow more space for the birth as the baby's head is crowning) are currently much lower than they were even five years ago. More and more doctors are being taught how to avoid episiotomies in medical school, and current research contraindicates them in many cases. Ask about the provider's induction rate and if active management of labor (AMOL) is advocated in his or her practice. AMOL is the practice of rupturing a woman's membranes, putting her on pitocin (a synthetic hormone that causes the uterus to contract), and giving her an epidural (a regional nerve block injected into the epidural space around the spine) in order to actively manage the progress of the labor.

How Long Has He or She Been in Practice?

Do you want a provider who has been practicing for years or someone new? New providers, fresh out of residency, have developed skills based on the most current research and are often more open to new ideas. On the other hand, they don't have the years of experience and wisdom of an older doctor, who may have delivered thousands of babies. Interview two or three providers before making a choice. This person will be a huge part of an unforgettable year of your life, so make the choice that is right for you.

Location, Location, Location

You also want to think about the environment in which you want to give birth. Aside from a hospital, depending on where you live you may have the option of a birth center. And of course there is always home birth.

Hospital birth is a first choice for many women because they want to be in a comprehensive medical environment, where, in case of an emergency, both mother and baby will receive immediate treatment. They also want to have all the available pain relief options. Most hospitals, unless they have a birth center, do not provide a homelike environment. Intervention is certainly more prevalent in the hospital than in a home or a birth center.

Oftentimes IVs are mandatory upon admission, women are not able to eat or drink, and their activity is limited. Not all hospitals have midwives available for labor and birth. Many hospitals have labor, delivery, and recovery rooms (LDR) in which women labor, deliver, and recover all in the same room. Gone are the days of whisking women down the hall on a gurney to the delivery room. Instead, delivery rooms are now used mostly in a high-risk situation.

In addition to hospitals, your community may have a freestanding birth center. Most of these centers have certified nurse midwives attending the births with physician backup. In a birth center or home environment it is much more likely that a woman will be able to move and change positions, as well as eat and drink during labor. A limited number of birth centers offer the option of water birth, which is considered by some to be the most noninvasive way to give birth.

You may be opting for a home birth. In this case it is imperative that you have an experienced midwife who has physician and hospital backup. There is probably at least one group of midwives practicing in your area. Interview them and check their references along with those of the backup physician.

You need to go into a home birth knowing that if your labor becomes high risk you will be taken to the nearest hospital. Medical insurance does not typically cover home birth.

Choosing a Hospital

There are several ways you can go about choosing a hospital. Sign up for the tour through the prenatal education department and see what you think. Ask friends, coworkers, and relatives in your community where they had their babies and if they were pleased with the care. Call the labor and delivery unit; if one of the nurses is free, you might have the chance to ask some questions. If you are in a community where you are able to choose among a number of hospitals, find the one that best meets your needs.

What Is the Hospital's Policy on Intervention During Labor?

Some hospitals have strict policies regarding hospital procedures, such as whether or not a laboring woman will require an IV. Some hospitals insist that a laboring woman have an IV from the moment she arrives; others require it only once active labor begins. Still others leave it up to provider discretion. In some hospitals you can be pretty sure you will be in bed for most of the labor; others encourage movement and walking.

Does the Hospital Provide Rooming In and Mother/Baby Care?

It is becoming more and more common for newborns to room in with the mother and go to the nursery only if there is a health problem. It is ideal to keep your baby with you, to enjoy skin-to-skin contact, and to get off to a good start with breastfeeding. Studies have found that babies who room in recognize the difference between day and night faster than babies who have been in the nursery. Some medical centers no longer have a newborn nursery for healthy, full-term babies; they all stay with their mothers. Mother/baby care is also becoming more common. This means that at the same time the hospital staff is providing immediate postpartum care for the mother, all newborn care and procedures (unless there is an emergency), such as weight check, bath, blood tests, and eye treatment, take place in the recovery room with the mother present.

Does the Hospital Have a Neonatal Intensive Care Nursery? What Level Is It?

A Neonatal Intensive Care Unit (NICU) is for the small percentage of babies who require special care after birth. The highest level of care is level three. If your pregnancy is high risk because of premature labor, or severe disease in the mother or the fetus, you may be transferred to a hospital with a level three intensive care nursery. If you or your baby have less severe problems, such as premature labor after thirty-four weeks, you may be transferred to a hospital with a level two nursery if that is closer to your home.

Are There Lactation Consultants on Staff?

Hospitals with a commitment to breastfeeding are likely to have at least one certified lactation consultant (CLC) on staff to work with new mothers. Before you go home, she will observe you breast-feed and help you with latch and positioning to make sure the baby is nursing well. If you are having problems she may recommend a breast pump or schedule you for a follow-up visit after you leave the hospital.

How Many People Can You Have in the Room during Labor?

You may want to have a "cast of thousands" helping you in labor. Make sure the hospital will allow you to have the number of people that you would like, though it may be disruptive to have them all in the room at once. You may have grand plans to have all your loved ones present, but then find once you are laboring that you want more privacy. There is typically a waiting area in labor and delivery for family and friends. Remember that if an emergency should arise, it is likely that all visitors will be ushered out of the room.

What Is the Nurse to Patient Ratio?

What is the nurse to patient ratio in the hospital? Will a nurse be taking care of you throughout the labor or will a "care partner" (a nonlicensed nurse's assistant) be tending to your needs? The nurse, as opposed to the doctor, is the provider who spends the most time with you in labor. If you are interested in having an intervention free birth, call the hospital in advance and ask for the names of the nurses who are the most supportive of intervention free childbirth. Keep in mind, though, that it is not guaranteed that they will be working when you go into labor and that not all medical centers allow you to request specific nurses. And, even if you can, their schedules may not permit them to be with you during your child's birth.

What Is the Doula Policy?

A doula is a person who has received special training in assisting a woman in labor. The word *doula* comes from a Greek word which means "mothering the mother." Doulas are typically women who have had a baby or have been closely involved with pregnant and birthing women. Some doulas volunteer their services, others run a professional service and charge a fee. Research has shown that having a doula can shorten the length of labor, decrease the requests for an epidural, decrease the cesarean rate, and increase bonding, maternal satisfaction, and the success of breastfeeding. Parents-to-be become concerned that having a third person present will detract from the intimacy of the experience, but for the most part having an experienced navigator helps diffuse the stress for both you and your partner. Find out if the hospital is open to doula support. Some hospitals have in-house doula programs, either on a volunteer or fee-for-service basis. You should also be able to get a list of doulas in your area from the perinatal education office at the hospital. DONA (Doulas of North America) also has a Web site (www.dona.com) with listings of doulas in the United States.

Is It a Teaching Hospital?

In teaching hospitals residents handle the majority of care during labor and birth. The beauty of this is that residents are up-to-date on research and procedures. Some women are very open to the concept of a resident. Others feel uncomfortable about having an unfamiliar doctor caring for them when they feel so vulnerable.

Are There Private Rooms?

Most labor rooms are private, although the triage area (the room you are taken to before being admitted) may be semiprivate. Most hospitals have private rooms for postpartum moms, though some of these may be semiprivate as well, meaning you will share the room with another woman. The private rooms are usually available on a first come first served basis. Your insurance may or may not cover this, so find out in advance.

What Is the Postpartum Visiting Policy?

How restricted are the visiting hours? Can family and friends visit even with the baby in the room? Hospitals in general are becoming less stringent about restricting visitors. Ask if there is a limit to the number of visitors you can you have in your room at a time.

Is There Adequate Security in Place?

Most hospitals have a security system on the maternity floor. For your own peace of mind you may want answers to the following questions.

* ✻ Does the staff wear color-coded badges indicating who can handle babies and who can't?

* ✻ What kind of security system is there in the maternity ward?

* ✻ Is there an alarm system and or a security guard on duty twenty-four hours a day?

* ✻ Are there security cameras? Is anyone allowed access to the area or is it restricted?

Pregnancy and the Workplace

You may want to speak with your employer in advance to determine how much freedom you have in changing your schedule to accommodate pregnancy and new motherhood. If you are lucky, you work with people who understand the need for flexibility at this time.

When Will You Share the News?

It is not too early to start thinking about what would be the best time to tell your employer and coworkers about your pregnancy. After exploring birth options, how will you balance your professional obligations with parenthood? When will you tell your supervisor and coworkers that you are pregnant?

> *Marlena, who had a management position in a hospital, waited until the end of her first trimester to tell her supervisor and coworkers that she was pregnant. She wanted to settle into her new reality before making others aware of it. Also, she wanted to wait until she had the results of her prenatal tests, specifically the amniocentesis. Knowing that there was a 20 to 30 percent chance of miscarriage in the first trimester also kept her from disclosing her secret in the first few months (see Chapter 2). If she lost the baby after everyone had rejoiced in her pregnancy, she feared it would be even more devastating.*

What about Disability and Maternity Leave?

For most pregnancies, the disability period begins four weeks prior to the due date and ends six weeks after a vaginal birth and eight weeks after a cesarean. If it is medically determined by your doctor that you are unable to work and you are under a doctor's care, disability may begin earlier in the pregnancy. When on approved maternity leave, women are also entitled to family leave as mandated by the government. The Federal Family and Medical Leave Act of 1993 allows a hiatus of twelve workweeks. Leaves taken under this act are generally unpaid, though it is required that your job be held until your return. Beyond that, you will need to negotiate with your employer.

Child Care Options

If you do return to work, what will you do for child care? Some couples work alternate schedules and are able to do the "hot potato" routine with their infant. It is wonderful for the baby to have both parents, but this can put a strain on the relationship because it is then difficult to eke out enough couple time. More and more workplaces are offering on-site child care, which is a wonderful solution for many new moms. They can nurse their babies throughout the day and spend the lunch hour with them.

If necessary, take the time to research child care facilities in your area. If your home and workplace are not in close proximity to each other, think about finding one that is more accessible from your workplace if that is where you will spend the bulk of your time. There are a variety of factors to consider when researching child care. Some of them are:

* How experienced is the caregiver?

* Is it a licensed center?

* Do they supply references?

* Can they accommodate infants?

* How many children and what age groups does the facility accommodate?

* What is the child to caregiver ratio?

* How close is it to your home or work?

* Are the philosophies of the caregivers similar to yours?

* If diversity is a priority for you, is it reflected in the children, staff, and activities?

* Will the child care providers respect and support your parenting choices, e.g., choosing to breast-feed or using cloth diapers?

* Is the facility clean?

* Will your baby receive enough attention?

* What are their discipline or redirection techniques?

* Are you welcome to spend time during drop-off or pickup hours?

* Can you interview other families?

* Is there an extra fee for arriving either early or late?

You may want to have someone come to your home on either a day-to-day or live-in basis to care for your baby. Consult the agencies in your community to help you find reliable, professional help.

You may be fortunate enough to have a relative or friend nearby who is willing to help you with child care. Of course, some women are faced with the sticky situation of having a less than ideal relative eager to take on the role of child care provider. You might choose to share in-home child care with a friend who has a son or daughter around the same age as yours. There are many creative solutions to the need for reliable child care.

Colleen and her neighbor Melissa had babies within two weeks of each other. Colleen worked part-time on special projects at the local university and Melissa grew organic herbs and produce, which she sold at a number of outdoor markets during the week. Neither of them had a need for full-time child care and they both worked unusual hours. But together they could provide one person with full-time work. They found a wonderful woman who was open to working for two families, sometimes caring for one baby, sometimes for both. This arrangement worked beautifully for them until the children were ready for preschool.

During your pregnancy your vision of the ideal life may include very few deviations from your work schedule and career goals. Some women are able to maintain their prepregnancy work schedule for the duration of their pregnancy and into the early parenting years. There may not be another choice financially, or perhaps a woman feels she can be a better mother if she maintains a career and outside interests. But after the baby arrives you may feel so concerned about leaving your child that returning to work seems physically impossible. You may feel suddenly resistant to relinquishing the role of primary caretaker to someone else. Also, you may not want to miss one moment of your baby's growth and development. Some women begin taking their babies to child care on a part-time basis before returning to work in order to wean themselves before leaving the baby full-time. The transition can feel much easier this way. Women who don't work outside the home or are in school may not need consistent child care, but may still be faced with making a part-time child care decision.

Maternal love is a powerful and often unpredictable force. Be prepared to have a number of unexpected feelings about leaving your baby once you become a mother. You might change your mind completely and decide to stay home full-time. Whichever path you choose at the outset, bear in mind that these choices are not irreversible and that throughout your years as a mother you may make a variety of decisions, professional and otherwise, that you would never have predicted.

In evaluating the practical decisions you have to make in preparation for pregnancy, arm yourself with as much research as possible. Having a wealth of information to draw from will allow you to make the wisest choices for this extraordinary period of your life.

Practical Considerations **Worksheet**

I need to choose:

☐ health insurance

☐ a health care provider

☐ a hospital or birth center

When choosing health insurance the things that are the most important to me are:

When looking for a health care provider the things that are the most important to me are:

When deciding on a hospital or birth center the things that are the most important to me are:

When considering a home birth the things that are the most important to me are:

The things that concern me most about returning to work and finding child care for my baby are:

6

Financial Considerations

Money is a volatile subject for most people. Those without it fear they will never have it; those with it fear losing it. Irrespective of their income bracket, some people are overwhelmed just imagining the financial impact a baby will have on their lives.

> *On her way to New York to visit family, Debra, who was thinking about becoming pregnant, began chatting with the woman seated next to her on the plane. As they spoke about their interests, careers, and relationships it became clear that this woman, a lawyer, enjoyed a lavish lifestyle. Still, when the conversation turned to having children, she said, "There's no way I can afford a child. Between child care, schooling, clothing, medical expenses, and extracurricular activities, I would go broke." Debra, a graduate student, whose partner was a struggling artist, came away thinking, "Boy, if she can't afford a child, what could I have been thinking?"*

How Financially Secure Do I Have to Be?

Some women feel a need to get their financial house securely in order before becoming pregnant. If this is the case you may find yourself opting to have a baby later in life, when you have established a solid economic foundation.

> *When Hilary was young her parents got divorced and she watched her mother struggle financially for years. As an adult she built a thriving career as a dentist and her husband, Jack,*

did equally well in his job as a financial analyst. Though Hilary wanted a child, she was not willing to compromise her lifestyle in the way her mother had. She did not plan to work full-time once she became a mother, yet wanted to maintain the lifestyle to which she and Jack were accustomed. She waited until she was thirty-eight and had a secure financial foothold before becoming pregnant. After James was born she returned to work three days a week and was able to devote the rest of her time to being a mother without financial worry.

Not all women feel the need to be this financially settled before becoming a mother, and it is certainly not a requirement for parenthood. Younger families who are not financially established are sometimes more willing to go with the flow and deal with issues as they arise, knowing that their financial situation will improve with time. Even if your financial situation remains less than optimum, you can still provide your child with a good education and many opportunities. Though this will probably demand more creativity and resourcefulness on your part. In many young families, one or both parents are in college, have not yet chosen a career, or have just begun their careers. In a sense, these parents grow up with their children.

Obviously if both parents work up until the baby arrives and then one stays home, they will have to adjust to a lower income level. For some people this is not a heavy burden. Some parents find themselves more than willing to scale back their lifestyle in order to spend more time with their child.

Chantal, an artist, continued to work at an art museum throughout her pregnancy. Her husband worked for a nonprofit organization. When her daughter was born she made the choice to be a full-time mother. Prior to parenthood they had been able to afford all the little extras—dinners at fancy restaurants, new clothes, vacations. They were now ready to forfeit this and focus on their daughter.

I'm Going to Spend *How* Much?

When considering parenthood, there is one thing that is indisputable—babies cost money. The cost of having a baby is significantly more than it was twenty years ago and continues to rise. Cesarean and neonatal intensive care unit (NIC) time inflate this cost. Certainly, this is not all out-of-pocket expense. If you have health insurance it should cover a major portion of it.

Some women are fortunate enough to receive health benefits from their or their partner's employer that include no-cost maternity care. If you have to pay a certain amount each month to your employer for coverage, it is obviously more costly. If you carry your own independent coverage, the financial impact of pregnancy and birth can be substantial.

Not all policies cover maternity care. You want to carefully review your coverage prior to becoming pregnant. In addition, there are policies that will not cover you if you are already pregnant. So, be careful about switching jobs and insurance plans while pregnant.

The current cost of raising a child to the age of eighteen is estimated to be $240,000 (after factoring in inflation). Housing and food are the two major expenses. Of course, clothing, education, and entertainment also factor in pretty heavily.

Although this is the time when you are getting acclimated, economically and otherwise, to providing for another person, the three years before school begins are generally the least expensive. Even this time, though, can be financially onerous if you have to pay for health insurance and/or child care if you and your partner are both returning to work.

What Your Newborn Will Need

Beware of advertisers trying to convince you that you need zillions of gadgets in order to successfully care for a newborn. Even in today's high-tech world a newborn's needs remain very basic. Naturally we want the best for our babies, but that doesn't mean we need to refinance our homes or become destitute in order to purchase all the newest items.

Newborns need to be fed, held, loved, changed, burped, bathed, rocked, talked to, and clothed. None of which are terribly costly. Babies don't care if the crib is lined with eyelet-edged gingham or if the stroller is the newest, state-of-the-art model. They need a place to sleep, a car seat, and a low-tech mode of transport, which in the beginning can be your arms, a front carrying pack of some sort, a stroller, or a carriage. If you can't afford a crib or bassinet, you could line a dresser drawer with bedding for the first several months and the baby would be just fine. Most people used to do this and many still do. The majority of items needed for a newborn are often handed down from family or friends, or can be purchased in fine condition secondhand. If your family members or coworkers give you a baby shower, you may receive many of the basic items as gifts.

Baby Basics

Despite many ads to the contrary the "must haves" for newborns haven't changed much. Although these don't have to be of the most expensive variety, it is critical that you use only those items that meet the latest safety standards. The costs for these items will vary depending on your location and style preferences. Certainly if they are purchased secondhand the cost will be significantly less. The baby basics are:

- ❊ A crib, cradle, bassinet (or safe place to sleep), which can cost anywhere from $60 to $600 depending on your specific preferences

- ❊ Bedding (sheets, mattress pad, blankets, crib bumpers), which can total between $130 and $300

- ❊ A car seat (hospitals require that you have one before they will release you with your baby), which costs a minimum of $80

- ❊ A carrier or sling (excellent for carrying and calming a newborn), which range from $30 to $80

- ❊ A stroller or carriage (for when the baby is a bit older), which will cost at least $60

- ❊ A swing (though not an absolute necessity, very useful for calming most fussy babies), which ranges from $40 to $120

- ❊ Diapers (ninety a week for a newborn), which total approximately $35 to $50 a month

* Clothing (T-shirts, pajamas, undershirts, one-piece cotton underclothes, socks, hats), each of which runs between $3 and $20

* Formula (if your are not breastfeeding) costs about $1,000 a year

A Word about Car Seats

If you depend on a car as your main mode of transportation, you want to make sure that it is safe and that there is enough room for an infant car seat. A two-door car can be a real struggle when you are routinely moving an infant and car seat in and out of it.

Unlike many other items, the car seat should be bought new rather than secondhand, unless you are absolutely certain that it meets current safety standards. The most common cause of death in children is car accidents, and sadly, many of those deaths could have been prevented by the use of approved car seats. *Consumer Reports* and the American Academy of Pediatrics give you the most current information regarding car seats for newborns. They are required by law in all fifty states.

Until the baby weighs twenty pounds and is a year old, car seats are designed to sit backwards in the center of the back seat. Medical centers, the highway patrol, and various private agencies offer car seat checks in which they ensure that they are installed properly and meet current safety standards. If you have two cars and can afford it, you may want to purchase two car seats for convenience sake. When the baby reaches twenty pounds and one year of age, you will need to switch to a bigger seat or adjust the one you have to its bigger size. Children are currently required to remain in car seats until they are forty pounds. A safety note: Use of the car seat should be a constant; your child should always be strapped in even if you are driving two blocks to the corner market.

Space: The Next Frontier

The accumulation of all these items leads to the next issue: Do you have enough room in your home for a baby? In the beginning a number of young families live in a one-bedroom apartment with their newborn, making the dining room, office, or laundry room into a nursery, or having the newborn share the parent's room. This can be a fine arrangement at the outset, but by the time the child is between the ages of two and five, it may become trying. If it is within their budget, many parents-to-be end up either moving or remodeling during the pregnancy or soon after the baby is born. The average price for a new house in the United States is currently $208,000. Families spend on average 21 percent of their income on housing. Bear in mind that our space requirements are specific to our culture. In many other countries families live in much closer quarters. It is all about what works for you and your particular lifestyle, how much spare room you have, and how you want to use it. Remember that a newborn's need for space is minimal, so in the beginning you don't want to be overly concerned about expanding your living space.

Staying Home

One of the most common questions prospective mothers ask is: "Can I afford to stay home if I want to?" More and more women are returning to work by the time their baby is three months old. Certainly that percentage has increased in the last five years. Some women don't have a choice—their income is necessary to keep the family afloat. You may, however, be in a position where your family can get by without your salary. In some cases you will need to scale back your lifestyle. There are women who are fortunate enough to be in a financial position that affords them the opportunity to stay home without impacting their lifestyle. In general, most new parents find they can get by with much less, particularly because their entertainment source has now taken the form of a newborn. Whether due to lack of finances or sheer exhaustion, you won't be making the social rounds in the beginning.

In considering the financial viability of staying home with a baby, you also want to consider what you would spend on child care. For some women, the expense of child care and the cost of travel to and from the daycare provider outweigh their monthly income, and for that reason returning to work is not the optimal choice. If the woman is the breadwinner of the family, she may be the one returning to work while her partner stays home. Some women have the option of working at home, and find that this helps them successfully juggle working and mothering. The decision to return to work or not is an individual one based on need and desire. More and more women are exploring creative solutions.

Your Money and Your Children

When it comes to their children, parents differ about how much money should be earmarked for them and when. Not all parents see the benefit of providing their children with a nest egg, believing that it is more to their benefit that they learn the value of earning and managing their own money. There are others, though, who want to do everything they can to secure their child's financial future. Some of the different ways in which parents view their financial obligations to their children follow.

❊ Some parents expect their child to be gainfully employed by age sixteen so they can cover their own personal expenses, particularly a car and car insurance.

❊ Some parents feel that their financial responsibility ends when their child turns eighteen. They expect the child to put him or herself through college without assistance.

❊ Some parents believe in setting up college funds for their children, but expect them to earn their own spending money while in school.

❊ Some parents support their child through college, spending money included.

According to current financial estimations, college costs rise 6 to 7 percent a year. There are Web sites that help you calculate exactly how much money you will need to save per month for your child's college. If possible, begin saving as soon as your baby is born.

The Big Financial Picture

Once you have worked through the short-term financial concerns, it's time to begin thinking about long-term financial issues. These include managing credit card debt; income tax; life insurance; setting up various savings accounts, trusts, educational and college funds; and drawing up a will. If your are not in the position to take on long-term financial commitments you might want to begin researching what some of the various investment and savings options are for the future.

Credit Card Debt

If you are carrying a lot of credit card debt or debt in general, it is a really good idea to clear it up before having a baby. It might be helpful for you to talk to a financial consultant about consolidating your debt.

Income Tax

Because a baby is considered a dependent your income tax status will be affected. Women who are due at the end of December usually keep their fingers crossed that they will not go past their due date so they will get a tax deduction before December 31. Talk to an accountant for detailed information about how a baby will change your tax responsibility.

Life Insurance

Life insurance is one of those things that many people don't think about until they become parents. Because it ensures that their children will be provided for if anything should happen to them, this investment brings peace of mind to parents. An insurance agent will be able to outline the costs and advantages of various plans. If you are lucky, your employee benefit package includes a good life insurance plan.

Saving Money for Your Child

There are numerous ways to save money, from piggy banks to tax-free educational IRAs. Educate yourself by reading money management books, attending financial management classes, or meeting with a financial consultant who can help you set things up in a way that best meets your needs.

It is not always the case that your philosophy matches your budget. You may have a strong desire to help your child financially but are unable to do so. Not all parents are able to set up trusts or savings plans for their children. When money is tight, it is easy to think, "We couldn't squeeze a penny out of our budget if our lives depended on it." You might be able to put only twenty dollars a month into an account for your baby, which doesn't seem like much, but over the years it will add up. If you are able to start even a little savings account for your child, you will not regret it.

Drawing Up a Will

In addition to meeting with a financial consultant, think about consulting a lawyer in regard to drawing up a will. At this point you might be thinking, "How morbid! Here I am thinking about having a baby and you want me to think about death." But planning for the future becomes much more important when there is a child in the equation. If you find yourself resisting this transition, try to think about it in terms of your child's life rather than your death. If your financial situation is simple at this point in your life and your assets are few, it is still important to have a will for the welfare of your child. Begin thinking about who you would want to raise him or her in your absence and make it legal. If your financial situation is complex and your assets are diverse, all the more reason to draw up a detailed will, once again with the welfare of your child in mind.

Be Ready for the Unexpected

Even with the best planning there are a number of unanticipated costs that will arise as you raise your child. Medical costs for children are always hard to gauge. By the time your child is school age you may find that your neighborhood public schools are not up to your standards, and private school tuition is considerable. Your child may end up with a passion for an expensive sport or hobby, which you want to support. And we cannot always predict the future of the housing market, our jobs, or our investments.

> When Maggie's children had both grown up and moved out, she did what many empty nesters do—she took stock of her life. She began to feel overwhelmed at how little she and Bruce had to show for themselves financially, compared to her sister Angela and her husband, who had never had children. One day she sat down and began calculating how much money she had spent on her children over the years. She jotted down some rough numbers from birth through age five for both of her children, which included doctor and hospital fees, diapers, child

care, preschool, clothing, furniture, housing, extracurricular activities, and tons of miscellaneous items. She threw up her arms in amazement once she finished, realizing that she'd spent more money than she ever would have thought possible. Despite the frustration she felt, she realized that having had the opportunity to nurture two fantastic children made her a wealthy woman.

Curtail the Retail

The one thing you are hopefully able to keep under control is your own spending. Your children are bound to have friends with parents who indulge their every demand for material items, and they will push you to follow suit. Families devise different strategies for dealing with their children's consumer demands.

Grace and her husband, both actors, live in Malibu, an affluent Los Angeles beach community with their two sons. By the time the boys were seven and eight their demands for material possessions and the amount of stuff that was cluttering the house had gotten out of hand. Grace and her husband did not want to raise children who took money and possessions for granted, and wanted to set appropriate limits. They decided to implement the following system: Once a month the boys got to go to the store of their choice to buy a new toy. It could cost no more than forty dollars and they each had to pay for half of it. They both did chores during the month, which gave them enough cash to cover their half. Instead of becoming impulse buyers, the boys really thought about what they wanted and valued the item after it was purchased. This system worked well for everybody and eliminated a great deal of conflict in the house.

Generous Gift Givers

Relatives, grandparents in particular, often cannot resist buying everything under the sun for their grandchildren. You should try to manage this early on so it does not undermine your philosophy on spending and gift giving. If they ask what type of gift they can give your child, you might want to request money or bonds (although you will probably have some relatives who would rather pick out gifts for your child). You can invest this for your child's future and it will go a lot farther than yet another trinket to add to the collection. Some grandparents like to begin saving or investing for the grandchildren, which can be a big help if the parents aren't yet ready to do so. Depending on their budget, some grandparents also like to buy the big-ticket items, such as computers. Others want to pay for education, vacations, or clothing. Some grandparents, particularly if they have limited resources, simply want to spend time with their grandchildren and go out for ice cream or a movie. This time together can far outweigh the value of any gift.

Use This Information to Your Best Advantage

You may be thinking, "I'm not even pregnant and here I am being encouraged to think about the finances of my distant future. How can any of this information apply to me?" Talking in such specific terms about the future can make you feel that you are being bombarded with information and encouraged to live for the future rather than in the present. But planning for your future financial security does not mean that you must abandon the present. Give yourself some time to absorb the information and, when you are ready, use it to your best advantage.

Financial Considerations Worksheet

In terms of my financial situation, I feel:

- ☐ Ready to become pregnant

- ☐ Like I need more time to put my finances in order before getting pregnant

- ☐ That even though I don't have much money now, I still feel like it's the right time to become pregnant

When my partner and I discuss the financial situation that we want to achieve before having a baby we:

- ☐ Have the same outlook

- ☐ Have a somewhat different outlook but are able to talk about the areas in which we differ

- ☐ Have very different outlooks but are able to talk about them

- ☐ Disagree completely and cannot have a reasonable discussion

- ☐ Haven't even talked about it

In terms of long-term financial goals that will benefit my children:

- ☐ I think about them a lot and have started making plans.

- ☐ I think about them a lot but haven't done anything yet.

- ☐ I think about them intermittently and have started making plans.

- ☐ I think about them intermittently and have done nothing yet.

- ☐ I haven't thought about them at all.

7

Your Changing Relationships

Perhaps you are in a relatively new relationship and already thinking about motherhood, or maybe you've been with your partner for years and coming to the "let's have a baby" turning point. You may be scrutinizing pregnant women and new families on the street, wondering, "Will having a baby really change my life and my relationships the way everybody says it will?" It is not uncommon to be fearful of the shifting dynamics that are brought about by pregnancy and childbirth. The familiar is always more comfortable, and after you have a baby life as you know it changes radically. Women often go through phases of planning for pregnancy and then reinvesting their efforts back into their everyday pursuits, because the thought of all the upheaval evokes such anxiety. Some of our ambivalence toward pregnancy is due to the changes it imposes on our relationship to others.

Making a Baby Together

For many couples, planning for pregnancy brings a new and vital energy into the relationship. The meaning of lovemaking changes, and intimacy often deepens with the intention of making a baby together.

> *After three years of marriage Maureen and Todd were ready for a baby. She went off the pill and the following month they were making love without birth control for the first time. The next day she reported to her friend Shelly, "I know this is going to sound crazy, but I think we made a baby last night. We made love in a way we never have. Thinking about making*

a baby together brought us so close. When it ended we both held each other and cried."

Maureen, like many women, had a sense about what was happening with her body. She was thrilled to discover that she had indeed become pregnant that night. Her only regret was that she and Todd weren't able to extend the fun and sexiness of the baby-making phase.

Not long after discovering she was pregnant, Maureen's body began to change. She had a difficult time adjusting to all the new sensations and feelings that seemed to multiply by the day. Two of her overriding concerns were, "Will I still feel attractive?" and "Will Todd still find me attractive?"

The Pregnancy Makeover

Attitudes toward a woman's pregnant body have changed significantly in the last twenty years. Women are increasingly able to maintain their beauty and personal style throughout their pregnancy. An ebullient pregnant woman is a beautiful sight that can turn heads on the street. For many women and their partners, pregnancy is a very sexy state of being. Demi Moore's seminude appearance on the cover of *Vanity Fair* gave us a collective opportunity to see the allure of a pregnant woman.

Veronica felt glowingly beautiful during her first pregnancy. She posed in the nude for her brother-in-law, a photographer, and felt suddenly glamorous and engaging. When out in public she wasn't surprised to find people looking at her admiringly.

Women certainly vary in their responses to their changing bodies. If the pregnancy is symptom free it is certainly more likely that a woman will feel more comfortable in her skin. Overall a woman's sense of beauty is redefined in pregnancy. It is no longer a static, image-driven beauty, but the beauty of creativity and new life.

While some women feel sensuously full figured, others feel fat and have trouble embracing their new look. A weight conscious woman might feel threatened by even a single pound of weight gain. Then there are those who feel betrayed by their body because for the first time they have no control over how it looks.

Counseling can help to resolve troubling self-image issues or difficult relationships with food.

Your Partner's Dilemma

Your partner may be unsure about how to respond to your appearance. Many men feel very attracted to the beautiful glow of their pregnant partners, but find themselves skating on thin ice when trying to express their admiration of it.

> *Heather and Richard were getting ready for a New Year's Eve party. Before the holidays Heather had purchased a lovely black velvet dress at a maternity shop, which she figured would get her through the party season. She was already dressed and putting on her makeup when Richard came into the bedroom and said, "Honey, you look so beautiful." She looked at him and thought, "Look at him—his body hasn't changed at all. Here I am, I can't fit into any of my clothes and he walks in like nothing's changed and tries to flatter me when I look horrible. He's just trying to make me feel better. He doesn't mean a word of it." She rushed to the bathroom and cried for a good twenty minutes. Richard spent the rest of the evening wondering what he did wrong.*

Not all women are this volatile or touchy during pregnancy. When it comes to how they feel about their normal bodies women are a diverse lot. Their feelings about their pregnant bodies are equally varied.

His and Her Worries

You might be one who watches other couples weather the storm of physical and emotional changes and thinks to yourself, "We'll never be like that." Preparing for the onslaught of the unknown feels like standing on the edge of a high dive looking down. Who knows what it might feel like to jump? The fall might be farther than you had calculated, the water might be freezing, and you might get hurt. On the other hand, the jump may be exhilarating beyond imagination, the water might feel great, and you might emerge from the experience with more confidence than ever.

Your relationship with your partner, your friends, your family, even yourself will all change as you prepare for and enter motherhood. Even if the pregnancy is physically manageable, you can expect a kaleidoscope of emotions during the nine-month period. You and your partner will be in the middle of a huge identity shift both within yourselves and with each other, which can strain even the most solid relationship. Men and women typically have their own separate constellation of issues that worry them. As they face the unknown together, prospective parents are nagged by a number of scary questions. Women usually ruminate on the following.

* Is my baby healthy?

* Will I make it through labor?

* Will my body ever return to normal?

* Will I be able to breast-feed?

* Will I be able to juggle career and motherhood?

* Will I be a good mother?

* Will I ever have time for myself?

* Will I be able to find good child care?

* Will I become just like my mother?

While men usually find themselves wondering:

* Will we ever have sex again?

* Can we afford a baby?

* Will we have enough money for college?

* How will I find time for my career and fatherhood?

* What about my own personal time?

* Will my child grow into a productive member of society?

* Will we have time for our relationship once the baby comes?

* What about sleep?

These differences in focus can in themselves be a strain on the relationship. A vulnerable pregnant woman and a fretful expectant father do not always make the most serene partnership.

Succumbing to the fear together can feel like being lost in the darkness without a guide.

Your Common Goal

Of course there is always an up side to every story. The fun and joy of getting ready for your baby is often exhilarating for both you and your partner. All the activity and new information enrich your life in a new way. You now have a project you are working on together, a common goal. You will find excitement in thinking about your baby and planning for the future together, in doing things such as:

* Lying in bed together and feeling the baby kick

* Comparing cribs at the local baby stores

* Decorating the baby's room

* Touring the labor and delivery area of your hospital and visiting the nursery

* Sharing your fantasies and visions with grandparents-, aunts-, and uncles-to-be

* Imagining your first night at home with your newborn

Before the Time Change

Time becomes an issue once the baby is born—time for the baby, time for your relationship, time for your family, time for yourself. What happens to all the time? Once you have a newborn you will see that the simplest tasks take twice as long. The day will go by and you will find it difficult to account for all the hours. It will be a struggle for both you and your partner to maintain a schedule and to keep up with self-nurturing activities. During pregnancy, while your baby is still in the low-maintenance phase, make the most of your private time. Do all the spontaneous things that you enjoy. Go on as many dates as you can, enjoy time with family and friends.

Share Your Concerns

A woman's response to her pregnancy has an impact on her relationship. Her partner may emerge as a champion nurturer, yet he may seem irritated or impatient at times. He may feel helpless and out of control about the dramatic physical and emotional metamorphoses taking place before his eyes. He also may be experiencing much of his own fear and worry that he will do his best to internalize in an attempt to keep you calm. It is important for both partners to have outlets for these feelings so they don't build up and become unmanageable.

It can have a polarizing effect if a woman and her partner do not communicate their fears and anxieties to each other. There is so much value in simply listening to and respecting each other's point of view. Sharing books about pregnancy, attending classes together, and journaling are helpful tools.

High Risk, High Tension

A difficult or high-risk pregnancy can cause even more strain. If a woman and her partner are used to being healthy and pain free, these changes can be very trying. In some cases a doctor will prescribe bed rest for a portion of the pregnancy, which can cause unprecedented stress in a relationship.

> *Wendy began having premature labor contractions in her twenty-eighth week of pregnancy. After his examination the doctor informed her that her cervix was already changing, and prescribed complete bed rest until her thirty-seventh week. Aside from some brief stints throughout the day, she could only get out of bed to take a shower, and would have to monitor her contractions daily. Her big outing would be going to her weekly doctor's appointment. Wendy, an architect, was in the middle of a huge redesign project and had planned to work as long as possible. Now she would have to consult via phone and hand off most of the work to her associate, which made her very depressed. She would have to discontinue her prenatal yoga class and set about finding a childbirth educator who would make house calls. In addition to his work as a city planner, Thomas, her partner, would be in charge of all the domestic duties. To top it off, sex was off-limits. They had a difficult*

time getting through this unexpected crimp in their plans. Fortunately, their friends helped out around the house and delivered meals to them. By the time Wendy was able to get out of bed, she was weak and exhausted, and Thomas was feeling overwhelmed. It took them a while to reconnect and stabilize their lives together.

Knowledge Trumps Fear

Women are often concerned that their partner, though tolerant of all the changes, will not understand them. It is helpful to attend childbirth preparation classes together. Typically, women are the ones who devour books about pregnancy. Men mostly get their knowledge from their partner's research or from the classroom. It is illuminating for men to see videos and charts detailing the physiological changes that take place in a woman's body. After all, these changes are hard to imagine.

Being in a classroom setting with others who are experiencing the same thing is comforting and often opens you up to new ideas and coping strategies. Classes on a variety of topics are offered in medical centers and in private settings by certified educators. Class topics include: early pregnancy, childbirth preparation, cesarean birth, VBAC (vaginal birth after cesarean), preparation for fatherhood, breastfeeding, newborn care, exercise, yoga, hospital tours, and infant CPR. Knowledge boosts confidence and decreases fear for everyone concerned. For partners, knowing the "hows and whys" of pregnancy, labor, and early parenthood facilitates greater understanding and empathy.

It is also recommended that your partner go to prenatal doctor visits with you. Hearing the heartbeat and seeing the baby's image on an ultrasound allows a father to share in the closeness that a mother-to-be has on a regular basis. Just lying in bed together, counting the baby's kicks and watching the baby undulate can be very sweet. Anything that can provide the father with a tangible sense of the baby fosters a greater sense of awareness.

Sex at a Time Like This?

All of these changes are bound to have an impact on your sex life. Women and men vary in their sexual desire during pregnancy.

Some women love their new bra size and feel ultrasexy. Since they are not worried about becoming pregnant because they already are, it feels liberating to make love without birth control. There is increased blood supply in the vaginal area, causing more sensitivity. Some women either experience orgasm for the first time, or begin having multiple orgasms.

If a woman feels unattractive she will be less inclined to want and enjoy sex. She may not want to be seen naked. Her partner's naked body, which used to thrill her, might now seem unappealing. Her breasts and tummy have grown and finding a comfortable lying position is challenging enough, let alone a satisfying sexual position. Certainly fatigue and/or nausea have been known to zap sexual desire. If you have had trouble conceiving or there has been any threat of miscarriage, the thought of arousal or penetration may make you fear for the baby's well-being. Or you may just become apathetic on the whole subject. It's also possible that you will find cuddling or various forms of touching more appealing than penetration.

This response can be difficult for a man who is wild about his partner's pregnant body. Her full breasts, ripe body, and the fact that she is carrying their child all culminate in a new level of attraction. If he is interested and she isn't, this can create tension. The reverse can also cause stress.

Some men feel worried that intercourse will stimulate labor, hurt the baby, or even that the baby will see what is going on and become traumatized. Unless a provider has prescribed "pelvic rest" (no sexual activity), it is important to remember that babies are quite safe and well protected in utero. The amniotic fluid that surrounds them acts as a shock absorber, the membrane around the fluid is quite strong, and the uterus is powerfully supportive. The layers of fat, muscle, tissue, and skin in the mother's body add an additional wall of protection. Though intercourse is often recommended as a labor-inducing strategy, it will not cause a woman to go into labor if her body isn't ready.

Toward the end of the pregnancy, standard positions, missionary for example, can become difficult for the woman and couples need to experiment with alternatives. The ones in which the woman controls the level of penetration are usually preferred.

It is not uncommon for colostrum (a yellowish fluid that the breasts produce prior to breast milk, which is high in antibodies) to leak from the nipples during arousal in the last month or two. Also, some women experience uterine contractions after sex and fear they are going into labor.

> *Marsha was in her seventh month when she and her husband Michael decided to spend a weekend out of town. He had been away on business for several weeks, and this gave them the chance to catch up and enjoy some of the quiet time they would miss when the baby was born. They had a wonderful time together, until, after lovemaking, she experienced low-grade uterine cramping. She remembered her childbirth educator saying that menstrual-like cramps could be a sign of premature labor. Frightened, she called her doctor back home who told her the cramping might be related to sexual activity. She advised her to drink several glasses of water, lie on her left side, and if the cramping persisted for over two hours, to call the local hospital. Within an hour the cramping was gone and Marsha relaxed, fairly certain that it was caused by sex.*

Some women enjoy a vibrant sex life up until the day they go into labor. As mentioned, sex is recommended by some care providers as a way to induce labor if you are past your due date. Intercourse, or any sexual activity that brings on orgasm, causes the uterus to contract, which may help promote labor contractions. There is also a labor-inducing hormone called prostaglandin in semen that might have some influence.

Not Our Mother's Pregnancy

Attitudes toward sex during pregnancy are often a reflection of the current cultural climate. Until the Sixties, women were cautioned against sexual activity for at least the last two, if not the entire nine months of pregnancy. Women were not as open with each other or with their doctors as they are today. Maternity styles often made women look like baby dolls rather than full-bodied women. Today's pregnant woman has the opportunity to look and feel glamorous.

And of course, childbirth was not a family event; fathers were not welcome in the delivery room. Rather, they were installed in the waiting room where they paced like caged animals. The only insight they had into the drama of childbirth was what their imaginations could conjure. The natural childbirth movement of the Sixties ushered in a new era—one in which men and women could celebrate the joy of childbirth together. Today not only are we able to speak more openly, but fathers are present for the birth, bringing them into the circle of inspiration from which they were previously excluded.

The Power of Mentoring

Educators hear of "office talk" about the negative impact that witnessing childbirth can have on a man's sexual desire.

> *When her baby was four months old, Sheryl called her child-birth educator because she and her husband had not yet resumed their sexual relationship due to his lack of interest. One of his office partners had told him how his wife's birth experience had turned him off completely. These comments had such a significant impact on Sheryl's husband that he was terrified to make love to her.*

In some cultures it is not traditional for a man to be with his partner during labor, possibly for fear that it will dampen his Hsexual desire for her. Also, there are women who view this as a uniquely female experience, which they don't want to share with their partners. Or they may simply fear that labor will cause too much stress for them. Even though it is now considered the norm for men to be present during childbirth, it is important for each couple to determine what works for them. There is no right or wrong.

Mentoring is a very powerful source of support for expectant couples and can often be a determining factor in how changes are perceived. Conferring with a man who has witnessed his partner in childbirth and emerged with a deeper connection to her and their newborn because of it can change the way a soon-to-be dad views this whole process.

Pregnant women, who are particularly sensitive to labor testimonials, can also benefit greatly from positive mentoring. It seems like in every checkout line there is a woman who tells war stories about her birth experience. It will only aggravate your fear and uncertainty if all you hear throughout your pregnancy are accounts of the pain and stress of labor and the problems that will arise in your relationship.

Self-Help

Certainly we all embark on this journey with our own emotional quirks and baggage, and positive mentoring might not be enough to guide you through the rough spots. Pregnancy and parenthood bring a lot of sensitive issues to the surface and you may find that counseling or self-help programs will help you gain perspective and insight. If you find yourself in need of extra support, you can get referrals from your care provider, friends, your spiritual counselor, or through various community agencies. You can choose individual, couple, or group counseling. People also find comfort in following a familiar or finding a new spiritual path.

The Facts about Domestic Violence

Because many of us envision pregnancy as a time of unparalleled joy and contentment, it is difficult to imagine that domestic violence could erupt at this time in our lives. The changes of pregnancy can induce stress and anger in a relationship and ignite a number of difficult feelings for both a woman and her partner. Violence crosses all boundaries—age, cultural, social, religious, and economic. It not only endangers a woman's life and well-being, but her baby is also at risk, particularly if she is struck in the abdomen. Also, with a violent parent in the house, it is more likely that child abuse will subsequently occur. Although violence is most likely to result from a male partner's alcohol or drug abuse, consistent or sporadic unemployment can also be a trigger. If you find yourself at risk for abuse, whether verbal or physical, it is critical that you ask for help. The National Domestic Violence Hotline offers confidential counseling and can be reached at 1-800-799-SAFE or via e-mail at: ndvh@ndvh.org.

A woman who chooses to leave an abusive relationship will likely feel most threatened by her partner right before and right after leaving. Generally, a woman is most compelled to take action when her baby's well-being is jeopardized. In order to protect her and her baby from harm, support is crucial, as is counseling or anger management for her partner.

The Changing Face of Friendship

Once you become pregnant you will, over time, notice a shift in your social life. Your relationships with single friends or couples without children will change. And why shouldn't it? Pregnancy causes a tectonic shift in the focus of your life and center of your identity. Inevitably, others will react. And this can set off a disquieting reaction of its own in you. Especially when close friends who do not have children begin to drift. It can also surprise you and bring you closer to certain people in your life. People's reactions vary depending on where they are in their own lives.

* Those friends and relatives who are used to having a one-on-one relationship with you might become jealous as you become more involved with planning for your baby.

* You may find that your relationship with certain coworkers was a "work specific" one and that once you are out of the work loop you have nothing in common.

* If you have women friends or family members who have experienced a pregnancy loss, or are unable to conceive, it may be heartbreaking for them to see you pregnant.

On the flip side of this shifting landscape is that you will certainly make lots of "mom friends." Pregnant women have a magnetic attraction for one another. You will meet in childbirth classes, in doctor's offices, in the park, at child care centers, in the baby store. Motherhood is the fertile common ground that will cause your bond to grow, and this new identity will stick for many years to come.

Me, Myself, and I

The relationship that probably undergoes the most sweeping change is the one with yourself. You'd be hard-pressed to find a journal big enough to record the myriad of emotions and reactions you will have during your nine months of pregnancy. You are overtaken by what one of my client's called "hormonal seismic activity." Women are often unprepared for the roller coaster that they suddenly find themselves riding. As the fetus develops, as your body changes, as your hormone balance shifts, your whole sense of who you are in the world gets reconfigured. This is both wonderful and terrifying. It is an opportunity for growth and expanding awareness, but as we already know, with change comes fear.

Pregnancy marks both an end and a beginning. An end of life as you know it, an end of a more carefree, open-ended life-style. Women often don't get the chance to reflect on this loss, particularly when the initial impact of pregnancy brings severe nausea, fatigue, or a more high-risk condition. Whether in therapy or not, women sort out many personal issues during pregnancy.

The Mother in Me

Your issues about your own relationship with your mother might surface during pregnancy. You might find as you approach motherhood that you are more like your mother than you ever thought possible. If you've begun the sifting process suggested in Chapter 1, you will likely find yourself thinking about the things your mother did when you were a child that you don't want to repeat. You might also begin to recognize and embrace the parts of your mother in yourself.

> *Nicole's relationship with her mother had never been easy. As a child she gravitated toward her adventurous, fun-loving father. She felt restless and hemmed in by the domestic world inhabited by her mother, and never made much of an attempt to understand her. As Nicole's pregnancy progressed and she began to see herself as a mom, she started to identify more with her mother for the first time.*

When it's all said and done, you may feel very positive about certain traits of your mother's that you see in yourself.

Like a New Language

Because it is impossible to experience these changes in advance, it can feel difficult to prepare. It is much like studying a new language. Before going to Brazil, you might immerse yourself in the study of the Portuguese language, but it will only come alive once you set foot in the country and begin to order in restaurants, ask for directions, and interact with native speakers. Not only will the language become real to you, but words will take on new connotations. Pregnancy preparation follows a similar pattern.

Educate yourself in advance so that you go into it with a certain degree of knowledge, but at the same time accept that there will be many unanticipated twists and turns in the road ahead. Lean into it—this roller coaster ride will be the first of many as you enter the world of parenthood and may well be a good working model for the rest of your life.

Your Changing Relationships **Worksheet**

When I think about being pregnant and how my body will change I am concerned that:

☐ I will not feel attractive when I am pregnant.

☐ My partner will not find me attractive when I am pregnant.

☐ Our sex life will change when I am pregnant.

☐ I will lose my sense of self while pregnant.

In order to cope with these concerns I will:

When I think about being pregnant and how my life will change I am concerned that:

☐ My friends will abandon me.

☐ My partner and I may have difficulty communicating.

☐ My relationship with family members will change.

☐ My relationship with myself will change.

To help me cope with these concerns I will:

I am concerned that my relationship with my partner might become abusive.

☐ Yes

☐ No

If yes, I plan to seek help by:

In order to help my partner be more involved in the pregnancy I will:

In order to help myself stay balanced during pregnancy I hope to:

8

Baby Care Decisions

When it comes to child rearing it's amazing how many people, parents and nonparents alike, have unshakable opinions that they will be all too eager to share with you. Strangers in restaurants will lecture you about the precautions you need to take in order to avoid spoiling your child; women at the bookstore will weigh in on the benefits of using cloth over disposable diapers. This input, solicited or not, can influence your decision making, but remember it is not gospel and should be taken with a grain of salt.

"So many decisions, so little time" could be the motto for pregnancy. Now that you are thinking pregnant, you will be making a host of parenting decisions. From conception on, each day brings new questions and challenges. Thinking about these issues in advance will give you the opportunity to make the best choices for you and your baby.

Breastfeeding

In many medical centers over 90 percent of women leave the hospital breastfeeding. But if there is no structured postpartum support, within two weeks this number drops dramatically, often by as much as 50 percent. Small nursing problems loom large in the middle of a sleep-deprived night, and women can lose confidence and abandon breastfeeding altogether. Some common problems after leaving the hospital are:

❃ Painful engorgement

✳ Sore nipples

✳ A baby who won't latch well

✳ Positioning of the baby that is not ideal

✳ Lack of confidence and/or knowledge

It is believed that because breastfeeding is natural, it is easy. It's true that just as some women's labors follow the textbook norm, there are those who breast-feed without a problem. For the most part, it is a shared learning process for both the mother and the baby. You, the mother, have the breast; your baby has a strong, dedicated suck. The two have never worked together before and both parties are learning via a sometimes scary on-the-job training program. It might take two to three extremely challenging and frustrating weeks to settle into a pattern.

Then somewhere between three weeks and a month things click and it becomes second nature. You clearly grasp the concept of ideal position and perfect latch, the nipples overcome the initial shock of ongoing contact with a voracious vacuum cleaner, and the supply and demand milk production system regulates itself. It is very rewarding for a mother to watch her baby grow and thrive, knowing that it is because of her milk. The most recent recommendation from the American Academy of Pediatrics (1998) is that babies receive exclusively breast milk, as opposed to artificial milk, for the first year of life.

Breast milk is always warm, always available, inexpensive and, by far, the healthiest food for your baby. It is full of antibodies and immunities, meaning breast-fed babies are sick less often. There is as much as a 60 percent decreased risk of ear infections; an 80 percent decreased risk of pneumonia; three to four times fewer cases of diarrhea; and an overall lower risk of asthma and allergies. The mother benefits from a decreased risk of both ovarian and breast cancer, and in the majority of cases, loses her pregnancy weight earlier. Breastfeeding a baby promotes a close bond between mother and child. Intuitively, it makes sense that the milk we produce naturally is better for our babies than a substitute.

Nonetheless, it is natural for a new mother to have at least one episode of panic in which she convinces herself that:

❊ She is not producing enough milk.

❊ She's never going to be able to hang in and get through the tough spots.

❊ The baby doesn't like her milk.

❊ Though she may be producing an adequate supply, the baby is not getting it.

❊ The baby needs a bottle of formula because the breast milk is not enough to satisfy his or her appetite.

If you have any of these concerns make sure to seek out consultants or specialists available in your community. Some childbirth educators and nurse practitioners specialize in breast-feeding support. Check to see if there are breastfeeding centers either at the medical center or in your community where you can get support, and, if necessary, rent or purchase breast pumps and accessories.

Regardless of how much research you do and how much advice you get while pregnant, a zillion more questions will arise once you have your baby. It is highly recommended that you and your partner attend a prenatal breastfeeding class, offered through your medical center or in your community. Your partner's support is a critical factor in your breastfeeding experience and will greatly influence whether or not you continue. Your partner can be the voice of calm and reason in the middle of the night when you have convinced yourself that the baby is starving or doesn't like your milk. There is not much that can compare to this support. It is also extremely important to choose a pediatrician or family practitioner who promotes breastfeeding and to have family and community support.

Shockingly, it's only in the last several years that it's become legal to breastfeed in public in certain states. President Clinton recently signed the Right-to-Breastfeed provision, which prohibits the use of federal funds to "implement, administer, or enforce any prohibition on women breastfeeding their children in Federal buildings or on Federal property." Carolyn Maloney, a Democratic representative from New York, who introduced the act stated, "Experts tell us that breastfeeding is an essential practice for ensuring infants receive the nutrients they need to develop. I am proud that the federal government is setting the standard of welcoming a woman's decision to breastfeed her child in our nation's capital and other federal property."

Bottle-feeding

Studies have shown increased incidences of respiratory infections, digestive disorders, diabetes, obesity, and ear infections among bottle-fed babies. Formula (pharmaceutical milk) is more expensive than breast milk and requires more preparation, causing a hungry baby to wait for a feeding. A bottle-fed baby's stools and spit-up have a much stronger odor than those of a breast-fed baby. On the other hand, partners or caregivers can readily feed the baby on their own without waiting for the mother to pump. The best reason to bottle-feed is if, after making an educated and open-minded attempt at breastfeeding, you determine that you or your baby are unable to do it.

Statistically only a small percentage of women are unable to breast-feed due to:

* Insufficient glandular tissue

* Insufficient milk production

* Severely inverted nipples

* A health problem requiring certain medications, which when passed through the milk will be harmful to the baby

* Previous breast surgery

Others choose not to for a number of reasons, such as:

* Breastfeeding is not condoned or supported in their culture

* Feeling uncomfortable, anxious, or self-conscious to the extent that nursing becomes a constant struggle

* Having a partner and/or family that does not support breastfeeding

Even if your baby gets two weeks of breast milk, that's two weeks of antibodies and skin-to-skin contact that he or she would not have otherwise received. Try in whatever way you can to overcome the barriers that might keep you from breastfeeding. Of course, in certain instances the baby is unable to breast-feed and requires a bottle.

If you do choose to bottle feed the baby, you will want answers to the following questions:

❅   What type of formula will I use? Premixed or dry? Soy?

❅   What brand?

❅   What type of bottle?

❅   What type of nipple?

Women are often under the mistaken notion that once they give the baby a bottle of formula, they have to stop breastfeeding. This is not the case. If, for some reason, pumping and storing milk is not possible while you are at work or school, you can breast-feed the baby mornings, evenings, and weekends and give him or her formula during the hours that you are away. Women of all occupations—firefighters, flight attendants, students, film agents, teachers, plumbers, actresses, architects, designers, and business executives—continue breastfeeding for a full year against all odds.

> *Kathleen, a flight attendant, visited the breastfeeding center with her two-month-old baby, Samantha. She wanted a pump so that she could get her baby used to taking a bottle before she began traveling again. She was scheduled to begin flying again in two months and though she was a dedicated breastfeeding mother, was resigned to weaning Samantha and starting her on formula at that point. The lactation consultant explained that it would be possible to pump and store an adequate supply of breast milk to leave with her husband each time she traveled, and that she could resume breastfeeding when she returned. This was a shock to Kathleen, who had no idea that she could utilize both feeding methods. It was also a great relief. She had been anxious about weaning her baby at such a young age and did not want to give up nursing, which she found so rewarding.*

If you do offer bottles to your baby, hold the baby in your arms as if you were breastfeeding. Hold the bottle yourself, do not prop it. This will ensure that the baby receives a regulated milk flow with minimal air, and helps you establish closeness and trust with him or her. You want your baby to associate a bottle with nourishment from mother (or father). People might say, "Why go to all that trouble of holding the bottle? Prop it for the baby—it will free your hands so you can do something else." But baby feeding time is sacred time—a chance for you to be close, regardless of the feeding method you are using.

The Diaper Dilemma: Will You Use Cloth or Disposable?

There are a number of reasons why people prefer cloth diapers. In general, they are less expensive than disposable, whether you use a diaper service or buy and wash your own. Many new parents prefer to have cotton against their newborn's skin, and believe it decreases the risk of diaper rash. Babies who startle easily may cry at the ripping sound when you pull off the tabs on disposables. Parents may feel that cloth diapers are less harmful to the environment than disposable ones. Others use them because it is part of their culture and it wouldn't occur to them to do otherwise.

> When Jennie visited her friend Yasemin and her new baby she was surprised to find her stirring a huge pot of boiling water filled with white cotton diapers. When she inquired about it, Yasemin explained "In Turkey, where I come from, this is what we do. It's what my mother and all my sisters did for their babies. We make our own diapers out of cotton cloth, rinse them out in the toilet, put them in a big pot, and boil them for hours until they are completely clean."

If you do choose to wash your own diapers, a bleaching product can leave a residue that can cause diaper rash. A hot washing machine kills bacteria. Some environmentalists say that cloth diapers are better for the environment because they don't end up in our landfills. Others say that professional diaper services use too much gas, water, detergent, and bleach, which is just as harmful. One of the most compelling reasons for using cloth is that you can always tell when the diaper is wet. The main way you know that your newborn is getting enough milk is by making sure you get six to eight wet and at least two poopy diapers each day—what goes in must come out. Because breast milk is not seen as it flows into the baby's mouth, it is not clear how much a baby is consuming, so an inexperienced mother could presume her baby is being adequately nourished when he or she is not. With the ultra-absorbent disposable diapers, it is sometimes difficult to distinguish a wet diaper from a dry one, making it more difficult to detect dehydration. Often you can't even tell the diaper is wet until the baby has urinated about four times because it soaks so deeply into the diaper layers. The good news is that the layer that's closest to the skin remains dry. But these diapers fail to provide important clues to your baby's health. Many educators recommend that parents use cloth diapers at least for the first three months when the nursing routine is being established, so they can be sure their baby is feeding well and not becoming dehydrated. A three-month gift certificate for diaper service or a supply of cloth diapers makes a great gift for a new family.

Many people go into parenthood wanting their choices to meet the high ideals that they have set. They want to do what is natural and healthy and are willing to spend extra time and even extra money to attain the highest assurance that their child will be healthy. But sometimes our babies don't easily accommodate our choices.

Sonia is a mother, who, out of concern for the environment and a desire to use only natural products, opted to use a diaper service for her daughter Alice. Her daughter was a very fussy newborn who cried incessantly. Sonia's mother suggested that her fussy granddaughter was uncomfortable with the feeling of a wet diaper and suggested they try using disposables to see if they could eliminate at least one cause of the crying. Lo and behold, they discovered that Alice was a baby who couldn't tolerate the feeling of being wet. The change from cloth to disposable made a tremendous difference both for Alice and her parents who were at their wits' end. However, it was difficult for Sonia, who was so dedicated to her beliefs. When she stood in line at her local drugstore with a box of disposable diapers under her arm, she couldn't help but feel that she was compromising her values. But she had to be flexible to accommodate her daughter's needs and to keep her family sane.

Some Common Concerns about Cloth Diapers

Most prospective parents have some reservations about cloth diapers. When trying to decide between cloth and disposable you may find yourself asking some of the questions below.

What If I Stick My Baby with a Pin?

New fathers in particular feel fearful about sticking their baby with a pin while diapering. They are usually relieved to learn that diaper pins have definitely become a thing of the past. New parents now use various types of metal and plastic diaper clips and diaper wraps with Velcro that go outside of the diaper.

Won't They Stink Up the House?

Since the diaper service provides a deodorized container in which the used diapers are stored this is not much of a concern.

Won't My Baby Feel Like He or She Is Wet All the Time?

Cloth does get wet, no doubt about it. You may find with cloth that you need to be a bit more diligent about changing your baby.

Won't Cloth Diapers Be Messier?

The diaper covers used these days are heavy-duty and have elastic legs. In general, breast-fed babies have looser stools, which create more of a cleanup job regardless of the type of diaper used.

Disposable Diapers

For some people, the convenience of disposable diapers outweighs any argument against them. Use 'em, take 'em off, throw 'em away—no laundering necessary. In general, though, disposables are more expensive than cloth. Certain babies develop skin irritation from the paper and plastic, and do much better with breathable cotton against their skin. Disposable diapers go into our landfills, and the plastic outer layer is not biodegradable.

When choosing a brand of disposable diapers for your baby, you will need to try different bands and see which shape fits your baby the best. It doesn't matter if you use so-called "boy" or "girl" diapers; there's not a distinct difference. Some parents compromise and use cloth at home and disposable when out on the town or on vacation. Be as flexible as you need to accommodate your lifestyle.

When cleaning your baby, it is preferable to use a soft baby washcloth with warm water or a baby wipe that is alcohol and perfume free, which is safer for your baby's skin. Then allow him or her to air-dry before putting on a fresh diaper.

Circumcision

Some expectant parents are relieved to learn they are having a girl because then they don't have to make the circumcision decision. Circumcision is thought to have begun in ancient Egypt for purposes of hygiene, but there is little evidence to confirm the relationship between circumcision and cleanliness of the penis. Attitudes and beliefs around circumcision have changed dramatically in the United States in the past twenty years. Until the 1970s the majority of newborn boys were routinely circumcised. Now parents want to make a conscious decision. There is no thorough data to help estimate the number of newborn males circumcised annually in the United States. The data provided by the National Center for Health Statistics (NCHS) estimates that about 60 percent of newborn males are circumcised, but this is thought to be inaccurate. It might be as low as 30 to 40 percent in certain communities.

The following are some common rationales for circumcision.

* In certain religious and cultural groups it is a traditional practice.

* Circumcised fathers feel it will strengthen the father-son bond if their sons look like them.

* People believe that it is easier to clean a circumcised penis, and that there is less risk of infection.

In most hospitals the pediatrician or obstetrician circumcises the baby within a few days after birth. Hospital policies vary: Some allow only the father, not the mother in the room during the procedure; others do not allow either parent in the room for fear they will become too upset.

Circumcisions done for religious reasons are done after the baby comes home. There are a variety of different clamps, the Gomco clamp, the Plastibell device, and the Mogen clamp that are used, and topical and or local anesthesia may also be administered. Although circumcision is a quick procedure it is hard to imagine that a baby wouldn't experience pain. An increase in both heart rate and blood pressure has been noted in babies undergoing circumcision. It is helpful if the mother offers the breast to the baby immediately after the procedure for comfort. The baby may fall asleep soon afterwards, which is a typical pain response for a newborn.

You will be sent home with special instructions regarding care of the circumcised penis, which will take several days to heal. Most of the complications that occur involve bleeding and or infection, and are minor. The results of two major studies suggest that the complication rate is somewhere between 0.2 and 0.6 percent.

Choosing Not to Circumcise

In 1989 the American Academy of Pediatrics, which once endorsed circumcision, altered its position. Several large studies have researched the risk of urinary tract infections and sexually transmitted diseases in uncircumcised males. The numbers cited were not significant and the academy changed its procircumcision stance. What is most important is that parents teach their sons how to properly clean an uncircumcised penis.

There are a number of reasons why parents opt against circumcision:

* In certain religious and cultural groups circumcision is discouraged.

* Uncircumcised fathers want their sons to look like them.

* After extensive research parents see no need to circumcise their boy.

* Parents do not want to subject their newborn to unnecessary pain.

* Fathers who were circumcised may regret it, and don't want to put their son through the trauma.

* It is a permanent, irreversible procedure.

Some grown men who were circumcised claim that it has reduced their capacity for sexual pleasure. In fact there are men who are having foreskin restoration surgery. When all is said and done, most parents make a decision about circumcision based on gut feelings. This can be difficult when the mother and father have different opinions. If this is the case, it would be advantageous to seek counsel from your obstetrician, pediatrician, or other support person in your community. It is important as you make these kinds of decisions to research both sides of the issue so you can come to an educated conclusion.

In its closing statement, with regard to circumcision, the American Academy of Pediatrics wrote:

> *Existing scientific evidence demonstrates potential medical benefits of newborn male circumcision; however, these data are not sufficient to recommend routine neonatal circumcision. In the case of circumcision, in which there are potential benefits and risks, yet the procedure is not essential to the child's current well-being, parents should determine what is in the best interest of the child. To make an informed choice, parents of all male infants should be given accurate and unbiased information and be provided the opportunity to discuss this decision. It is legitimate for parents to take into account cultural, religious, and ethnic traditions, in addition to the medical factors, when making this decision. Analgesia is safe and effective in reducing the procedural pain associated with circumcision; therefore, if [the] decision for circumcision is made, procedural analgesia should be provided. If circumcision is performed in the newborn period, it should only be done on infants who are stable and healthy.*

Where Will Your Baby Sleep?

Where a baby sleeps is a very personal family choice. Some babies sleep in cradles, some in bassinets, others in cribs. Some share beds or co-sleep with their parents. Many cultures throughout the world sleep in family beds, often because they do not have the space for separate bedrooms, nor the luxury of central heating. There are varying points of view surrounding the "where will the baby sleep?" question. People may tell you:

* It is psychologically harmful for a baby to sleep with you because he needs his own space in order to develop properly.

* You might roll over in the middle of the night and smother the baby.

* If a baby sleeps with you she will become spoiled and dependent and will never leave your bed.

* If a baby sleeps with you, forget about ever having a sex life again; he will be sleeping between you and your partner forever.

* If a baby awakens in the middle of the night, you should go to the baby's room instead of bringing her to your room. This way she will identify her room, not yours, as her sleeping place.

As with all new parenting advice you receive, consider the source and try not to overreact to these warnings. Keeping a baby in your bed can be nurturing for everyone in the family. Do your own research by reading baby books and speaking to child development specialists, your pediatrician, and friends who are parents and have viewpoints you respect.

When Michelle was eight months pregnant with her first child and in the process of putting the nursery together, her father sat her down and said, "It is critical to your baby's psychological health that she have her own room and sleeping space." Michelle heeded what she thought was sage advice from her father and proceeded to assemble the nursery. When Clara was born she and her husband Seth put her in a bassinet by their bed, figuring that in two months' time she would move to her crib in the nursery. As it turned out, Clara was a fussy baby who really liked to be close to her parents, and as the days wore on Michelle found that bringing her to bed in the middle of the night facilitated the nursing/sleeping cycle for everybody. Cuddling with her baby was so satisfying, and Michelle could also offer her breast on demand while she and Seth snoozed through feedings. However, each time she had Clara in the bed she wondered if she was doing the right thing. At two months she moved Clara to her crib, and when she would awaken in the middle of the night Michelle was reluctant to

take her into bed with her. Her father's warning had made her
distrustful of her maternal instincts.

All it takes is for one alarmist to grab your arm in a Toys 'R' Us aisle to fill you with fear about ever inviting your baby into your bed. Babies love and thrive on skin-to-skin contact. If they had their way most of them would spend all day in your arms, or better yet in your bed, naked, right smack next to you. This doesn't mean that you have to sleep with your baby if you are not comfortable with the idea. If you are inclined to have your baby in bed but worried because of all the negative press you have been exposed to, remind yourself that each family makes personal choices and what works for your sister might not work for you and your family. In making your choice you do want to consider the latest recommendations regarding decreasing the incidence of SIDS. Soft bedding and particular sleep positions are thought to increase the risk of SIDS. The current recommendation of the American Academy of Pediatrics is that healthy infants, born at term with no medical complications, be placed down for sleep in a nonprone position. On the back is preferred, but the side is also considered to be safe.

Won't I Spoil My Infant?

There are differing philosophies about responding to babies around sleep issues, but the prevailing one is that it is not possible to spoil a newborn. Infants are motivated by instinct and do not yet understand cause and effect. They do not lie awake at night thinking, "If I cry loud enough, turn bright red, and make gagging noises, that nice mommy with the warm milk will come feed me."

It is important for you to respond to your baby; this is the way she learns trust. It is also important to find a system that works for you. You may put her to sleep in her crib or bassinet at the beginning of the evening but after two or three feedings find that taking her into bed with you is much easier, and that you get more sleep that way. It may be that having the cradle or bassinet next to your bed feels close enough for you. There are also co-sleepers that fold down and connect to the bed so that your baby is right next to you, but you each have your own space. If your baby is a particularly noisy breather or fidgets in his sleep, it may not be comfortable to have him in bed with you or even in the same room. It may also be that, with the baby next to you, you worry more and it disrupts your sleep. One thing is for certain, whatever routine you set up in the first two weeks will change by week three. It generally takes at least two to three weeks to build a relationship, understand the baby's cues and find your own stride. If you have a second baby you may find that what worked with the first is very different from what works with the second. Keep in mind that nothing is written in stone—try to be as flexible as possible during this trial and error period.

In general, most new parents keep the baby in their room, either in a bassinet, cradle, or in their bed. Some parents feel comfortable with the baby in another room if they have an intercom system. The "where will the baby sleep" question is often influenced more by the mother's feelings than the baby's.

> *Donna and her husband, Paul, lived in a one-bedroom duplex until their daughter Ana was five months old, at which point they moved into a two-bedroom duplex. For the first five months Ana had been sleeping in a bassinet next to her parents' bed. When they moved she began sleeping in a crib in her new bedroom. She transitioned from bassinet to crib without a problem. Donna, on the other hand, had trouble sleeping with Ana on the other side of the house. After the second night she wanted to move the baby back into her bedroom, but Paul convinced her that Ana was fine. It took Donna a good month to acclimate to the separation.*

Will I Ever Make the Right Decisions?

As a woman considering pregnancy you may feel ill equipped to make all of these life decisions for your baby. Just thinking about so many of them can feel overwhelming and the stakes feel so high. You may feel compelled to read everything you can get your hands on and/or solicit advice from everybody you meet. And still comes the gnawing doubt, "One misstep and I will traumatize my child for life." We all want to do the right thing as parents, and everybody has a different opinion of what that right thing is. In addition, people are not shy about giving new parents advice. Remember, research and input are valuable, but at a certain point go with your instinct it is usually a very reliable source.

Baby Care Decisions **Worksheet**

In thinking about whether I will breast-feed or bottle-feed my baby I think I will choose:

☐ Breastfeeding

☐ Bottle-feeding

☐ Both

Because:

In thinking about whether I will use cloth or disposable diapers I think I will choose:

☐ Cloth

☐ Disposable

☐ Both

Because:

In thinking about whether I will circumcise or not circumcise my son I think I will choose to _____ .

Because:

In thinking about where the baby will sleep I think I will choose_____ .

Because:

In thinking about what kind of bed my baby will sleep in I think I will choose _____ .

Because:

9

New Baby, New Stress

We have learned that the physical, hormonal, and emotional changes of pregnancy can at times feel like you and your partner have suddenly taken off on a wild roller-coaster ride. Though some women discover a newfound sense of well-being, this is not universal. In fact, women's responses are as varied as women themselves.

Once the baby moves from the in utero low-maintenance phase to the in-your-arms high-maintenance phase, a new level of stress is introduced. The day you walk through your door cuddling your newborn, you cross a threshold in more ways than one. It cannot be overstated: Having a baby is a sweeping life change. Too often we fail to consider the monumental effect that becoming a new parent will have on our lives.

Did Somebody Say Sleep?

Following birth, the physical recovery and fatigue are draining. By the second week postpartum, when the effects of sleep deprivation have kicked in, a new mother's tolerance is put to the test.

Sleep deprivation is disruptive to say the least. In certain countries it is used as a form of torture when prisoners are under interrogation. They are allowed to fall asleep and then awakened repeatedly, until they confess. This is not dissimilar to what a newborn does. Just as you fall into a deep sleep, you are awakened by his or her unrelenting cry. In the first two months it is almost impossible to awaken refreshed. When new parents talk about their lives, they universally begin by saying, "If only we could get a good night's sleep ..."

> *Rochelle and her boyfriend Curtis were invited to speak at their childbirth educator's class. They told their birth story, after which they were barraged with questions about parenthood. Somebody asked them if they had been able to find any time to spend alone together or make love since the arrival of their child. Curtis responded, "If we have the choice between cleaning the house, having sex, and sleeping, sleep comes first without a question, cleaning comes second, and lovemaking comes in a distant third."*

Consistent lack of sleep colors your worldview. New mothers and their partners become impatient, ill tempered, frustrated, and even despairing—all these feelings and more at a time when you want to be exuding positive energy for your new baby. Certainly there are variables in how a new mother deals with lack of sleep. Some women cope with it better than others. Also, some babies sleep more than others.

The Cry Baby Blues

The cry of an insistent infant can disturb a sleep-deprived mother's nervous system so profoundly that she feels her blood is boiling. It can take weeks for a new mother to learn to interpret her baby's cries and know the difference between an "I'm hungry" and an "I'm tired" cry. It takes weeks, sometimes months, for a new mother to learn that it is okay to let her baby cry at times and that she needn't rush to his aid every time he whimpers. However, remember that crying is the last indication of hunger, so you don't want your baby's "I'm hungry" cry to go unanswered. Until a mother is comfortable with encouraging her baby to practice self-soothing techniques, she will most likely experience agitation when her baby is crying. A new mother will experience a range of responses to a crying infant. It's not the crying alone that causes stress, but the emotions that the crying elicits. You may react in any of the following ways:

❋   Become extremely anxious and overwrought

❋   Break down and sob in frustration with your crying baby

✳ Become angry and resentful

✳ Become frightened and worried

✳ Lash out at your partner and cast blame

✳ Become withdrawn and depressed

✳ Lose confidence and think you are doing everything wrong

✳ All of the above

Some mothers are able to maintain their cool while the baby cries, but it seems universal that every new mother has her breaking point. What can you do for yourself when you hit your limit? What can your partner do for you? How will you remain calm in the face of all these new feelings? Who has the presence to remain calm when their baby is shrieking?

From where you sit these questions probably sound like no-brainers. Even experts in child care have noted that they were confident in their parenting know-how until they had children of their own. It is easy to come up with confident answers in advance. You may have already thought some of the following:

✳ Give the baby a pacifier.

✳ Let the baby cry him or herself to sleep, it's not a big deal.

✳ Hand the baby over to the father—he'll stay cool and calm.

✳ Call a relative to come help.

✳ Leave the baby with your partner, friend, or relative and go take a walk.

✳ Call a girlfriend.

✳ Take a hot bath.

✳ Put on some music.

Theoretically these all sound plausible, even realistic. But when your baby is squawking and you are exhausted, having a maternal meltdown seems far more likely to occur before any of the above does. In fact, recognizing that you are overwrought, overwhelmed, and overcome by exhaustion and anxiety is the only way to go. Being a postpartum mother and taking the enlightened path aren't always compatible concepts. So you're going to have to cut yourself some slack and give yourself some time before you master the art of remaining calm while your baby hollers.

> *When Angie and Joe brought their daughter Melissa home, it was alarming to see how different real life was from their fantasies. Melissa was a tightly wired, fussy baby who was very difficult to soothe. Her crying not only worried Angie, who had so wanted to be the perfect mother to the perfect baby, but also caused her to become angry with her daughter. This anger, combined with the baby's temperament, introduced a level of stress into their lives that they had never experienced. Joe could see that they were caught in a swirl of stress, but didn't know how to relieve it. Getting through each day for Angie and Joe was like managing raging rapids.*

Some of the recommended solutions to a new mother's dilemmas are fairly simple. Taking time out is usually a big help. Anything a new mother can do that is just for her, even for ten minutes, can make a difference. Once there is someone who can stay with the baby, taking a walk in the park, on the beach, or anywhere in nature can be very refreshing. For some women shopping is therapeutic. Hot bubble baths are wonderful. Naps are delicious.

It is nearly impossible to eliminate the sources of stress— we cannot make a baby stop crying or eating. We cannot decide one day to stop changing diapers. We cannot wave a magic wand and make our baby sleep through the night. We cannot decrease the laundry load. We cannot shut the door to the nursery at five in the evening and say, "See you tomorrow." So, how do we stay on top of all these tasks and duties while remaining calm?

Your partner can be a godsend by being attentive and picking up the slack in whatever area it is needed. Partners are really good at just about everything, including baby bathing, diaper changing, burping, holding, meal preparation, laundry, and house cleaning—actually, everything but breastfeeding.

Divvying Up the Domestic

Who does what around the house, anyway? The workload in the house will feel as if it has doubled once you bring the baby home, and division of labor can become a hot issue. Who does the laundry? Who makes the money? Who spends the money? Who cooks the meals? Who spends more time with the baby? Who changes the diapers? Who cleans the toilet? Things that seemed benign in a relationship prior to your becoming parents can become the cause of intense friction.

More often than not, both the mother and partner are working outside the home in addition to managing all the domestic chores. There is a lot of variation in the way couples divvy up household duties. Some couples, prior to the woman's becoming pregnant, share the workload, so it is no big deal to continue in this spirit. Some work through these issues during pregnancy and come to a comfortable compromise. Some men who have never even boiled water have a crash course in cooking during pregnancy, especially if their partner ends up on bed rest. Some men are the clean freaks in the house and it's the women who need to take Organization 101 in order to meet their standards. Some working couples choose to hire domestic help so neither of them has to do the chores.

In a household where two parents are splitting tasks, what is a reasonable expectation? It seems fair to imagine that each person will do 50 percent. The question is: Fifty percent of what? It may not be realistic to expect that each person will do half of the diaper changing, half of the laundry, half of the cooking. Certainly if a mother is breastfeeding she is doing more than 50 percent of the feeding. This ideal often does more to increase stress than to alleviate it. The splitting of tasks often comes down to who has the most stamina for which job. As long as everybody is pitching in, it's probably better not to waste precious energy measuring who does what.

The Postpartum Roller Coaster

In the past ten years focused research has been done on postpartum mood changes and stress responses. Statistics indicate that 80 percent of new mothers in our society experience some degree of postpartum depression. In its mildest form you feel blue and have fleeting tearful episodes. This may last an hour, several days, or perhaps a month or two. Some women, though, lapse into severe depression that is not remedied by the usual self-administered pick-me-ups. They most often require counseling and or medication to regain their equilibrium.

Stacey called her childbirth educator when her baby was two months old and said, "I think I had an episode of postpartum depression yesterday. I got in the shower and cried the whole time. Then I got out and felt fine." For Stacey, this was her one brush with postpartum depression and though it sounds equivalent to a light sprinkle, to someone with Stacey's temperament it may have felt like a hailstorm.

When Autumn was six weeks postpartum, her concerned husband, Rob, called their childbirth educator with a laundry list of worrisome symptoms: "She seems pretty depressed. She'll barely get out of bed and really isn't interested in the baby. She's not eating very much. She cries a lot, and I can't get her to talk to me." Their educator suggested that, as a first step, Rob get Autumn out of the house and take her to the park or the beach. She told him that along with everything else, women can get a bad case of cabin fever after giving birth. Autumn was exhibiting some very clear symptoms of postpartum depression. Rob took her to the beach that afternoon, which cheered her up considerably. For the next week they went on an outing every day and by the end of the week, Autumn was feeling about 75 percent better. For her, being in nature was the key to regaining her sense of balance.

Alice, who was forty when she had her first baby, was a list maker. Everything in her life ran according to a tight schedule and nothing was left incomplete. She considered herself efficient, organized, self-sufficient, and responsible, as did her employer. She worked until the day she went into labor. Throughout her pregnancy, she ate well, exercised, and gained the perfect amount of weight. Her labor was lengthy but once she had her epidural she slept until she had to push. Although she was exhausted after the birth, for about the first ten days she was upbeat, chatty, and thrilled with her baby. Then, at about two-weeks postpartum, without warning, she shut down. She cloistered herself in her bedroom, and wanted nothing to do with the baby. In addition, she stopped eating and sleeping. Her husband could hear her weeping from the other side of the house. He tried everything he could to motivate her, but nothing worked. After four days he called her obstetrician for advice and was referred to a psychiatrist who put her on antidepressants. Alice had a long road ahead of her, but the medication did a great deal to lift her severe depression.

Other extreme postpartum conditions, such as postpartum psychosis and postpartum panic disorder are uncommon, though they certainly occur. Postpartum psychosis is characterized by hearing voices and obsessive thoughts about hurting the baby. The signs of postpartum panic disorder, also rare, are severe anxiety symptoms: inability to sleep, heart palpitations, and shortness of breath. This can often be a result of a traumatic birth experience.

Seventeen years ago, Dasha gave birth to a daughter. Her labor began with her water bag breaking and progressed smoothly until she was about nine cm dilated. The baby was in a posterior position and because Dasha had a fairly small pelvis, she would not descend. After fifteen hours of labor she had a cesarean. During the surgery the spinal anesthesia moved upward into her chest and she could not feel herself breathing. Since the anesthesiologist did not take the time to explain that this was a side effect of the medication, she was sure that she was dying. The surgery itself went smoothly and her daughter was healthy and robust. About three weeks after the birth, Dasha began having anxiety symptoms. She slept fitfully and would awaken with a pounding heart; it felt like an engine was running at full speed inside her. She couldn't swallow, and sometimes thought she might die. At times it felt like she was going crazy and, worse yet, it seemed like all the new mothers she met were coping so much better than she. When she reached out to other women who had had babies, they all acted like the transition to motherhood was no big deal. She called her childbirth educator, who, despite her expertise, had very little information on postpartum syndromes. Turning to her book collection, Dasha hoped that one of them would have a section on postpartum emotions. She found one line in one of her books that mentioned "free-floating anxiety" and was mildly reassured that this is what she had. The anxiety persisted and she finally sought counseling. Her therapist, a warm, compassionate woman, never once suggested that it might be the aftermath of birth trauma. It took years for Dasha to recognize that she had had a severe case of postpartum panic disorder.

Today, Dasha would hopefully have a very different experience. There are now a number of good resource books available, as well as hot lines and support groups in many communities. Childbirth educators are more informed and knowledgeable and there are compassionate counselors specializing in postpartum conditions. Luckily, there are also medications available that can help a woman through the tough spots. Dasha still would have experienced sleep deprivation and the feelings that accompany the transition to motherhood, but she may not have felt so isolated and overstressed.

Where Does the Time Go?

Time becomes a greater issue once a baby is born—time for the baby, time for your relationship, family time, time for yourself. What happens to all the time? Once you have a newborn you will see that the simplest tasks take twice as long as they once did. The day will go by and you will find it difficult to account for all the hours. It will be a struggle for both you and your partner to maintain a schedule and to keep up with self-nurturing activities. During pregnancy, while your baby is still in the low-maintenance phase, make the most of your private and relationship time. Do all the spontaneous things you enjoy. Go on as many dates as you can, enjoy time with family and friends. Once your baby is born your time will be occupied caring for him or her. Time management becomes a coveted skill for new mothers, particularly when returning to work. If you aren't good at it now, your baby will be a marvelous teacher.

It is hard to imagine the number of hours a newborn will demand.

* Breastfeeding mothers spend sixty to seventy hours a week feeding a baby.

* Your baby will be awake, wanting your attention, at least twelve hours a day.

❊ You will change approximately ninety diapers a week; each changing requires time and attention.

❊ It will take you at least an hour longer to do just about any basic task.

❊ Each time you leave your house you will be packing your diaper bag with enough paraphernalia to sustain you through a month-long European tour.

❊ You will lose track of time, and time as you know it will cease to exist.

Am I a Good Mother?

A newborn's temperament has a large impact on a new mother's ability to cope. There are those babies who cry only when they need something, are equipped with self-soothing skills, digest food easily with minimal discomfort, and seem to feel calm inside their skin. If you get a baby like this, it is a breeze to feel confident about becoming a new mother—it's almost as if the baby walks you through the transition. Then there are the more time-consuming babies, the ones that are fretful and possibly colicky. These babies are tense, difficult to soothe, and often are not capable of soothing themselves. It can be hard to read their cues. A fussy baby is much more work and can create a lot of anxiety for the new mother. When a new, already anxious, mother gets one of these babies it can further undermine her confidence because it seems like nothing she does makes it better.

> Marla, the mother of a two-month-old demanding baby, felt envious of her friend Elaine. Elaine's son Sam cooed often, cried little, nursed well, and seemed so content. By contrast, Marla's daughter Grace was fidgety, colicky, and shrieked often and for no apparent reason. Her feedings were fragmented and she experienced frequent tummy aches. Marla felt it was somehow her fault, that if only she could be a relaxed mother like Elaine her baby would be perfect.

These feelings are typical for a new mother. Most new moms think that everybody else has it together, that they are the only ones feeling edgy and out of control. The smooth sail into motherhood is a myth, though it is true that some women just have an easier transition than others. The reasons for this run the gamut. It can depend on a woman's birth experience and her feelings about it; the temperament of both the mother and the baby; how much support a new mother has; her readiness to be a mother; her feelings about being at home with a newborn; how well she copes with lack of sleep; and her breastfeeding experience. And this list is by no means exhaustive.

> *Julie was put in a double postpartum room after having a long labor, which culminated in a cesarean. She was exhausted and in no shape to hold or take care of her daughter. Her roommate Anna was on the other side of the curtain cuddling her new baby, Jonathan. Unlike Julie, Anna had had an uncomplicated vaginal birth and was now enjoying her baby. As Julie lay in bed, fighting back tears, she could hear Anna falling in love: "Jonathan, oh my little boy, hello sweet baby, Jonathan, I'm your mommy, hi there." Julie wanted nothing more than to hold her baby and coo and cuddle, but knew she just wasn't up to it.*

Had the staff been more sensitive they would not have put these particular women in a semiprivate room. From the outset, Julie's fears about not being a great mommy were aggravated, and this led to feelings of discouragement and guilt.

There is a tendency for some mothers to become very competitive with others about whose baby sleeps through the night first, cries less, smiles more, turns over, sits, or crawls before the others. This competition burdens a new mom with even more stress. Each relationship with a newborn is a unique experience. It is helpful to understand infant development overall, but even more important to understand how your baby is wired so that you can respond in the best way possible. Babies are not cookie cutouts; they require individual understanding and management.

Flexibility is a winning trait for a new mother, as babies' needs and patterns change often and without warning. But going with the flow can feel exceedingly difficult for someone who is accustomed to a very structured or achievement-oriented life. Breastfeeding is based on demand feeding, which means feeding the baby according to her hunger cues rather than a schedule. Life with a newborn is pretty much about getting "nothing," according to normal standards, done. It is a stretch for some women to consider the accomplishment in endless diaper changes, feedings, baths, and holding sessions. Time becomes very open-ended and it can feel like you're not doing anything. Implicit in this lifestyle is the need to be flexible. If you live for your lists, how are you going to survive these first months with your newborn?

On the flip side, it can be a challenge for a free-spirited mother to give up her freedom to the demands of a baby. By two months most babies have moved into a more or less predictable nap schedule and your life will revolve around both his eating and sleeping habits. Your spontaneous spirit will take a backseat to the baby's needs and schedule.

Assemble Your Tool Box

Coping skills that reduce stress and increase well-being can make all the difference. Before becoming pregnant, find a stress management tool that works for you, such as yoga or meditation, and add this skill to your new mother repertoire. Managing stress has become a lifetime pursuit for many in today's chaotic world. People of all ages and occupations seek refuge in books, audio and videotapes, lectures, workshops, and retreats.

The skills that are the most effective have their foundation in the deep breathing you will learn while preparing for labor and birth. Deep abdominal breathing relaxes the central nervous system, decreasing the production of stress hormones known as catecholamines and increasing the production of endorphins, a natural morphine that the body produces, which translates into a greater sense of well-being. Meditation, yoga, martial arts such as tai chi, and biofeedback all have their roots in deep, slow breathing and use the breath as a tool to stay focused and in the moment, taking things one breath at a time.

Meditation

Here is an example of a stress reduction meditation you can implement in your life. You can do this as a lying down, sitting, or walking meditation. It relies on concentrating on the breath coming in and going out, quieting the mind, and focusing on the moment.

1. Sit cross-legged on the floor or on a floor cushion.

2. Lengthen your spine as you drop your shoulders and loosen the muscles in your neck.

3. Let your hands fall gently into your lap, opening the palms upward, releasing tension in your arms and hands.

4. Gently close your eyes.

5. Breathe slowly and gently in and out of the abdomen. Count to five slowly with each inhale and exhale. Use the breath to bring your attention to the present moment.

6. Let your body relax, allowing muscles to release a little more with every exhale.

7. Quiet your mind as you breathe. If thoughts interfere, clear your mind, letting them come and go like clouds passing in the sky.

8. With each breath simply repeat a word such as "now" or "peace" or "breathe" in your mind.

9. Breathe relaxation into your muscles and breathe tension out. With each inhale feel calm come into your body. With each exhale feel tension and distraction release.

10. Allow all the muscles in your body, from your head down to your toes, to release and relax.

11. Stay focused in the moment.

12. With a clear mind, visualize an image that you find calming. As you continue to breathe deeply with relaxed muscles, focus on this calming image, and use it to help you relax even more.

You can use this technique anytime you feel stressed or anxious; simply sit still, breathe deeply, and quiet your mind.

Relaxation Techniques

Some women prefer to learn stress reduction in a classroom setting, others read books or use audiotapes. There are numerous techniques available. Here are examples of some of the different methods you might want to research:

❊ Progressive relaxation: Lying on your back, relaxing the muscles in the body systematically from the head to the toes

❊ Touch relaxation: A partner facilitates the progressive relaxation of muscles from the head to the toes with gentle touch

❊ Neuromuscular dissociation: Alternate tensing and releasing of muscles in your body, from the head to the toes

❊ Visualization and imagery: Clearing the mind and replacing stressful thoughts and images with those that suggest tranquility and relaxation (flowing water, flowers, sunsets, beaches, etc.)

As you try these methods for yourself you will find that some work better for you than others. It works best to have a dedicated time each day to devote to practice. For some people sitting still and breathing deeply works beautifully; for others, visual images are very effective. Practice these techniques and discover which ones are most effective for you.

What else can you do to alleviate stress? There may be a variety of programs available through your local community center, gym, YMCA, church, synagogue, adult education program, community college, or private studios. They may offer meditation classes, tai chi or yoga classes, stress reduction seminars, or weekend retreats. If these types of things aren't available, perhaps you can be the one to start a program in your area. Other things you might try are:

❊ Walk twenty to thirty minutes a day.

❊ Take a dance, exercise, or aerobics class.

❊ Put on music at home and exercise or dance for twenty minutes a day.

❊ Use an exercise, dance, or yoga video at home.

❊ Swim.

❊ Take a personal half hour each day to nurture yourself.

❊ Take a bubble bath.

❋ Write in a journal.

❋ Sit and sip a cup of tea.

❋ Read a book.

❋ Get a massage.

❋ If you are at work, close your office door during the lunch hour and sit quietly, listen to classical music, or listen to a relaxation tape.

❋ Mix and match techniques to create your own version of self-care.

What will you do with your baby while you take care of yourself? There are activities you can do with your child, especially as he or she gets a little older, that can meet your stress reduction needs as well as provide a fun activity for the baby. Find places that offer child care while you swim or exercise. Take your baby out in a jogging stroller or in a bike tent.

The more internal housecleaning you do prior to becoming pregnant, the more relaxed you can be during your pregnancy and the postpartum period. The more practiced you are at these new techniques, the more likely they will become natural responses. This means that when under stress you will be able to readily access them. When you find a method that works for you, not only will it reduce your own personal stress, but the overall stress level of the household.

Don't Wish It Away

It is tempting for a new mother to wish she could transcend the strain and drudgery of the present moment: "If only she would sleep through the night." "When he starts eating solid foods, life will be easier." "I can't wait until she is older and she can tell me how she feels." *Don't wish it away*, is one of the best pieces of advice for a new mother. The newborn phase flies by in a blur and suddenly your baby is college bound. It sounds like a cliché, but the years go by quickly and babies stay in the delicious newborn phase for a very limited time. In seeking your own stress-relieving tools, think about how you can best help yourself remain in the here and now with your baby. Whether you are breastfeeding, changing a diaper, folding laundry, or giving the baby a bath, remember that this particular moment with your baby will not happen again. If you punctuate each moment with, "If only . . .", "When will he . . .", "Why won't she . . .", "I can't wait until . . .", you will be missing out on the wondrous experience before you.

Humor Yourself

Whether you are thinking about pregnancy, are newly pregnant, are in the final months of pregnancy, or are a new mother, remember to maintain your sense of humor. Humor, an essential ingredient for surviving parenthood, is the thing you might lose first as you set your intention on becoming pregnant, particularly if you have waited a long time to have a baby. Thinking pregnant can become such serious business that you forget to laugh. Try to see the lighter side of life as you begin this journey, despite any disappointment or pressure you may feel. Laughter is one of life's greatest antidotes.

The More Tools the Better

There's no getting around the fact that once your baby arrives, your boat will be knocked off its course. Your baby comes into the world with a unique disposition and you may find yourself at your wit's end trying to control his or her temperament and schedule, or trying to interpret various cues. What you will be able to control are your own responses to the unanticipated stresses of motherhood. The more tools you have under your belt in advance, the more likely you will be to keep your cool when the newcomer rings the bell.

New Baby, New Stress Worksheet

In order to decrease my stress, I usually:

When I think about being a new mom some of the things I worry about are:

☐ Losing sleep

☐ Losing my sense of humor

☐ Having less free time

☐ Having a fussy baby

☐ Not being able to juggle all the new tasks

☐ Having trouble being flexible

☐ Not feeling like a good mother

I worry most about the following:

The reasons I worry about these issues are:

To help me meet these challenges I will:

10

Dads

Expectant fathers now have unprecedented access to pregnancy and child-rearing information and support. Classes, books, television and radio programs, Web sites, and support groups designed exclusively for dads are now part of the parenting landscape. The old model of the father as an emotionally remote breadwinner is becoming obsolete. With an increased sense of confidence and awareness, dads are becoming more involved in the pregnancy decision, the pregnancy itself, and child rearing. Not only are they actively included in the birth, but they participate in infant feeding, diaper changing, and bathing, and some of them even become the stay-at-home parent.

Once a woman becomes pregnant, visits to the doctor, classes, family gatherings, and social interactions focus on her—and rightly so. After all, she is the one turning green with nausea in the first trimester. She is the one with the lower back pain or heartburn; the one whose body is visibly expanding. She is the one who feels the baby kick and swim; the one who will go through the awesome experience of labor.

Men, on the other hand, awaken to the same body every morning of the nine-month pregnancy and, unless they experience sympathetic discomforts (some men experience something called Couvade syndrome and have sympathetic symptoms like nausea and fatigue during the pregnancy), have a pretty easy time physically. This is not to suggest that they do not experience the full range of emotions during the pregnancy, from bubbling excitement to abject terror, and men are not always encouraged to share their feelings. At a family gathering while the women are engaged in personal conversation about the emotional highs and lows and discomforts of pregnancy, an expectant father's cousin or uncle might take him aside, raise his eyebrows and ask, "So how many times have you been sent out for weird food in the middle of the night?" or "Guess sex is a thing of the past, eh?" Though this may be a bit of a caricature, it is not typical for men to engage each other in deep conversation regarding their feelings and responses to pregnancy.

This has led in some instances to the mistaken notion that men do not experience these feelings. Because they do not express them does not mean they are not present. It can be extremely illuminating for both partners to explore in advance the range of emotions an expectant father might go through during the pregnancy. It will surely enhance future communication. Although, let's not forget, pregnant women are and need to be fairly self-focused. In most cases they will not have the wherewithal to worry too much about what their partner might be going through.

So, What Might He Be Going Through?

Do men go through a sifting process similar to the one described in Chapter 1 when preparing for fatherhood? If so, how do their issues differ from those that women face? Though certainly not a rule, in general, men tend to worry about different things than women. Their "Am I Ready" list might look something like this:

* Am I financially stable enough to be a father and provide for a family in the way that feels adequate for me?

* Am I ready for my sex life to change?

* Am I ready to assist my partner during labor?

* Am I ready to share my partner with a baby?

* Am I ready to forfeit my freedom?

* Am I ready to be the kind of role model I want to be? (This question can be especially pressing if a man has had a troubled relationship with his own father or mother.)

✳ Am I able to live up to the image I have of my own father, who was the greatest dad?

✳ Am I ready to take on the responsibility of raising a morally sound child who will be a contributing member of society?

✳ Am I willing to take time away from a demanding job to spend time with my child?

These questions might knock around in a guy's mind literally for decades before his coming to the conclusion that he is indeed ready. In biological terms men have a different time frame than women. Whereas women are born with a limited number of eggs, men continue to produce sperm throughout their lives. So, particularly ambivalent or free-spirited men may tell themselves, "What's the rush? When I'm ready, I'll become a father." While a woman's biological mantra becomes, "Gotta have a baby now, gotta have a baby now," a man's continues to be, "Take your time, take your time."

When they first moved in together Charlotte and her partner, Jay, agreed that within a year they would start trying for a baby. When the year anniversary rolled around, Charlotte, age thirty-six, was eager to get started. Jay, by contrast, was as ambivalent as Charlotte was eager. He didn't feel ready to be a dad, and had a hard time seeing how he could balance the demands of fatherhood with those of all his other interests—there just didn't seem to be enough hours in the day. Charlotte was torn between wanting to be understanding, as Jay had been about her ambivalence to move in together, and the urgency she felt about having a baby. It seemed as if her body was screaming, "Now, now, now!" Jay, on the other hand, acted like they had all the time in the world.

Of course, there are situations in which a man is ready for a baby before his partner. There can be any number of reasons why this might happen. Perhaps the man is older. Maybe the woman is involved in her career to the degree that motherhood would be too disruptive. Maybe she is scared to relinquish her independence. Maybe she has doubts as to whether this particular relationship will be able to withstand the stresses of parenthood. There are so many things that need to be in place for a couple to make a conscious decision to have a baby, it does seem amazing that two people ever say "yes" at the same time.

Making More Than Love

Men, like women, experience lovemaking differently once the intention of making a baby is in place. How long it will take for a woman to become pregnant is up for grabs. Couples might hope for an extended period of time to enjoy sex and might become pregnant on the first try. For other couples, there can be a great deal of anxiety if it takes too long. If it doesn't happen on the first try, some men find themselves reconsidering and waffling a bit. "Maybe I'm not as ready as I thought I was" and "Maybe we should wait a little longer" are not uncommon sentiments among men in this situation. Some become agitated and want things to happen immediately; others are very patient and figure there's no reason to stress, it will happen soon enough.

Now That She's Pregnant . . .

Once a woman is pregnant a whole new set of emotions kicks in for a father-to-be, once again ranging from bliss to terror. He may be the one who wants to stand on rooftops and call out the news to the entire world, while she wants to keep the news under wraps until she has gotten through the first trimester. He may feel a quiet excitement that builds as the pregnancy progresses.

During the first trimester, before a woman is showing, it is often difficult for a man to grasp the reality of the pregnancy. He might not really tune into the fact that his partner is pregnant until the tail end of the pregnancy or even until after the baby is born. It is not uncommon for a man, as the baby's head is crowning, to exclaim with wonder, "Look, we have a baby!" As if for the first time he realized that this would be the end result of pregnancy. It is nearly impossible for a man to identify with the physical changes a woman experiences while pregnant and his response might remain one of denial, even with the obvious statement made by her ever-expanding tummy. Men range in their level of involvement for a number of reasons.

When Margie, who is admittedly a big planner, was in her sixth month of pregnancy, the nesting urge hit her. She wanted to get the house ready for the baby, which included buying furniture for the nursery. Her husband, Thomas, seemed almost indifferent, and she felt like she was dragging him around town from one store to the next. She took his response personally and felt that he didn't care, that she was the only one invested in the pregnancy. His lack of enthusiasm and participation created a lot of anxiety for Margie during the pregnancy. Months after the baby was born she was able to see that Thomas had in fact been very excited about the baby, but that his way of processing change was very different from hers.

From the moment Willa and her husband, Rafael, witnessed the positive result of the in-home pregnancy test together, Rafael was brimming with excitement. He invited his family and closest friends for dinner that weekend and made an announcement. Each shopping trip became a reason to buy something for the baby—a pint-sized baseball cap, a book, a piggy bank, a mini football. He did everything he could to make Willa more comfortable while she was pregnant, including attending all doctor's appointments and prenatal classes with her. Sometimes, especially when she was experiencing heartburn and back pain, it seemed to Willa that he was more excited than she was.

There are a number of ways that you can encourage your partner to connect with the baby during pregnancy, such as:

* ✻ When lying in bed at night, put his hand on your tummy to feel the baby kick (if your baby is a junior gymnast, he may feel the kicking just lying next to you).

* ✻ He might enjoy singing to the baby, regardless of whether he can carry a tune. He might even write a personalized composition for your little one.

* ✻ If he is a music lover, he can play music for the baby.

* ✻ He might take a more literary approach and read to the baby.

* ✻ He can just improvise and talk, tell jokes, or family history to the baby.

All of these suggestions can make a significant difference in the way he interacts with the pregnancy and the baby. Make sure he knows that, at birth, your baby will recognize his voice. This will bolster the connection he feels.

A Great Source of Support

Fathers-to-be can be the greatest source of support for a pregnant woman. They can do numerous favors that can lift you spirits, such as:

* Go out at midnight in the pouring rain for French fries or other salty snacks

* Massage your back or tired, swollen feet at the end of the day

* Run a warm bath for you

* Give you positive feedback about your changing body, e.g., never using the word "fat"

* Cook dinners for you and wash the dishes

* Clean the house or have the house cleaned

* Paint or wallpaper the baby's room

* Bring you flowers without there being an occasion

* Sing to the baby

* Read to you

* Plan a vacation or weekend getaway before the baby is born

Will I Be Any Good at This?

When the second trimester kicks in, as the baby is more evident and the birth more imminent, fathers-to-be might begin feeling more concerned and fearful about the impending changes. Two of the questions that nag at most expectant fathers are:

* Will I be a good role model?

* Will I be a good provider?

Becoming a Role Model

Some men have had wonderful relationships with their fathers and feel confident that they can duplicate their parenting success. Others do a great deal of self-exploration about their relationship with their own father or mother, particularly if it was a difficult one.

Maurice had very little respect for his father who had divorced his mother when he was sixteen, following a string of affairs. After the divorce, his father was married and divorced three more times and had affairs during those marriages as well. He had been caught up in his own drama for most of Maurice's childhood, and had basically been a nonparent. Maurice prided himself on being a faithful, dedicated partner to Rona. But when she became pregnant he felt a current of fear that when he became a dad he would repeat his father's behavior.

When Earl's wife, Betsy, became pregnant, instead of feeling the excitement that he had been counting on, he felt a sense of unshakeable dread. He wasn't able to identify what was going on until he had a heated phone conversation with his mother in which some difficult feelings from childhood resurfaced. A few days later he was able to tell Betsy that he was worried, that, as a parent, he would repeat his mother's controlling behavior to the detriment of his child's psychological health.

Being a Provider

Men vary in how they define the term *provider*. For some of them it means being the sole breadwinner in the family. For others it means carrying most of the financial load, but not all of it. Some think providing 50 percent of the household income is sufficient. While still others feel fine about letting their partner bring home the bacon. Certainly there are situations in which the woman has a far greater earning capacity than the man, and it makes more sense for her to return to work after the baby is born. There are countless ways a family can balance the workload of both caring for a baby and maintaining financial security. In the interest of not just being a good provider but a good father, some men change careers or go back to school. They seek out jobs or rearrange career goals so they will have more time to be an active, participating parent.

> *Len had been working as a baker for ten years when his wife became pregnant. He worked long hours and had some job-related physical problems. Though he often thought of a career change, he had been reluctant to act on it because he felt comfortable with his work, made a decent salary, and couldn't really imagine what else he might do. He enjoyed sports, but didn't see the possibility of a career for himself in the field. As he thought about becoming a father he realized that he wanted to feel less physically drained and to be assured that he could have more time to spend with his child. Much to his surprise, an opportunity came up for him to be the program coordinator for a sports organization. He accepted and soon after the birth of his daughter, changed careers.*

> *Vincent's job in the environmental services department of a medical center provided him with only a meager salary. Still, he had many interests and hobbies outside of work that he managed to pursue. His wife, Caroline, was a corporate lawyer, who enjoyed much greater pay, and loved her work. In thinking about child care and all the juggling they would have to do after Caroline returned to work, it occurred to Vincent that he could be a stay-at-home dad, which proved the perfect solution.*

A Father Has Feelings Too

There are so many feelings an expectant father might experience. He might feel:

* Excited about all the wonderful things that are happening

* Ill at ease with the physical changes of pregnancy that he cannot identify with

* Left out and ignored

* Jealous of the attention his partner is getting and of his partner's relationship to the baby

* Mystified by how quickly things are changing in his life

✻ Exhausted by the needs of his partner

✻ Eager to become a father

✻ Stressed about dividing his loyalties and time between work and home life

✻ Concerned about the changes in his intimate relationship and sex life with his partner

✻ Scared about the idea of caring for a baby, e.g., changing diapers

✻ Anxious about how his relationship with male friends might change

✻ Worried about having less time for himself

✻ Scared of not being the perfect, supportive partner and father

✻ Concerned that he has limitations that may put too much of a burden on his family

✻ Worried about his ability to be a good role model

✻ Unprepared for the whole thing

Some of these feelings are easier to talk about and manage than others. Sharing joy and excitement usually comes easily for most couples. The way men express their emotions ranges from barely perceptible to over-the-top. And in some situations the woman is more apathetic than the man about the whole event. In these relationships it is the man who ends up dragging his partner to prenatal classes.

When it comes to a couple's emotional interactions in pregnancy it's hard to generalize. Some women are fairly self-sufficient, others like to be pampered. Some weather the changes calmly, while others feel mired in anxiety and confusion. Men's reactions to this are also highly particular. There are those who have no problem slipping into the role of nurturer and caretaker. They participate and listen, and are as eager to give feedback as they are a foot massage.

But when the man is anxious and overwhelmed himself and his pregnant partner is feeling fragile it can be a trying time. Where will he get the strength to be the bulwark of the entire family? Whom does she lean on for support and affirmation? Who does he lean on for support if he is taking care of her? These issues become more pronounced in cases of high-risk pregnancy, particularly if the woman is on bed rest and in need of ongoing physical assistance. A situation such as this, in which the health of the baby, mother, or both is threatened can arouse a great deal of fear for a man. It is unthinkable in many cultures and social circles for a man to stand up and admit to feelings of fear or helplessness. It is practically a taboo response. Again, who does he lean on? A woman has an ongoing relationship with her care provider, which likely gives her a sense of comfort. In addition, she is often sharing concerns with other women, both relatives and friends.

Jealousy

Jealousy is probably one of the more challenging feelings that expectant and new fathers experience. Admitting fear is one thing, but admitting to feeling jealous of an unborn or newborn baby seems downright selfish. Why do these feelings arise? A pregnant woman elicits a great deal of attention from both friends and strangers. If the man enjoys being at center stage, he may find this disconcerting. Also, she is very much in her own world, wrapped up in thoughts and feelings about her new body, giving birth, and becoming a mother. Subsequently, a man can feel left out of the mother-baby duet. If he is used to being babied and pampered by his partner, the sense of loss can be profound. It is helpful for a woman and her partner to recognize in advance how common it is for an expectant and new father to burn with jealousy about the mother's bond with the baby and the lack of attention he is getting. If a man is unable to allow himself such feelings, he is more prone to acting out. Men who feel left out and ignored do a number of things to avoid confronting these feelings. They may work long hours, stay out late with friends, drink, take drugs, have affairs, sulk, or become emotionally remote.

> *Nicoletta and Charlie's baby was a week old and she was still recovering from a difficult cesarean birth. Charlie, a workaholic who traveled extensively, was due to go on the road in two weeks. Nicoletta was still housebound and not up to much, so she stayed home with the baby when Charlie went*

out. One day he came home much later than anticipated. When Nicoletta, exhausted from caring for the baby on her own, questioned him, he admitted that he was having an affair.

Obviously having an affair when a woman is recovering from birth is not a productive way to express hurt or anger. This experience injected a lot of mistrust and stress into Nicoletta and Charlie's marriage, which might have been avoided had he been able to admit his feelings of abandonment and hurt.

The reverse is also possible. There are some situations in which a new dad becomes so enamored of his baby that the mother is the one who feels jealous and excluded.

In Support of Dads

Historically fathers have not had much support available. Luckily, today, there are various outlets for an expectant father who is feeling overwhelmed. A man might choose one of the following options or take advantage of all of them.

Classes and Support Groups

Some communities offer classes for expectant dads, which supply a lot of valuable information not only on the practical matters like how to burp and diaper a baby, but also on child development, pregnancy, relationship concerns, and parenting techniques. In prenatal and childbirth preparation classes, the focus is on the pregnant woman and growing baby. This leaves men with very little opportunity to voice their concerns. In a class or group designed specifically for them, they have a supportive forum in which to express their emotions. Being in a group of men who are experiencing similar feelings and insecurities translates into greater insight and confidence.

Journaling

Keeping a journal during pregnancy is a productive way for an expectant father to process feelings and alleviate stress. Not all issues need to be raised in a group or couples setting. Some fathers keep journals that are exclusively personal; others fill theirs with entries addressed to the baby. They share hopes and dreams with their unborn child in a way that is very meaningful. Max wrote daily during his wife's pregnancy. Here are some of his entries:

> *October 11, 1996*
> *Jesse is two months along and we've told almost everyone. It's a relief to have others share the knowledge and excitement. Jesse says she feels like Homer Simpson, "Donut ... Must have donut," and someone who has suddenly lost some physical ability. Whenever she comes home with another grocery bag full of junk food she says I shouldn't let her go out by herself. She's also talking about all the cute things she sees for kids in stores, and I'm starting to think about a second job.*

> *December 5, 1996*
> *Three months and counting. Lots of wild, vivid dreams lately. A full spectrum of emotions, actions expressed in them. This morning I woke up from one in which we had determined to name the baby Yokuradon. Scary!*

> *February 27, 1997*
> *Last night was our first Preparation for Childbirth class. The class is a real cross section of Bay Area unions. Only one straight, Caucasian couple, several mixed race pairs like us, and one lesbian couple. The first lecture was about the stages of labor and was fairly informative. It was the first time I got the sense of what an incredible ordeal it is. I have the sense that Jesse will handle it well, that being informed and having some stress management techniques will give her the tools she needs to cope. Another interesting point was about the nesting instinct—that for women it's about home and for men it's about working and making money. I'm not sure if that's not what I would be feeling anyway given that our house is still under construction and our budget is strained. At least we'll be in our own home soon.*

Counseling

Either individual or group counseling can help a father-to-be through the tough times. Some men feel devastated by the issues that come up during pregnancy and are unable on their own to put things in perspective. A therapist or counselor can be instrumental in helping men identify issues and resolve internal conflicts. If a man has had a terrible relationship with his own father, perhaps he will be able to find some peace before the birth of his own child. We all have a lifetime of learning ahead of us, and internal housecleaning is helpful, if not essential, before leaping into the world of parenthood, a world replete with new issues and challenges.

Bonding in the Birthing Room

Many new fathers claim that the initial contact they have with their child in the birthing room is the glue that bonds them together. Often the nurse will hand the baby to the dad for the first cuddle during the immediate recovery period, while the mother is being cared for. It is recommended that a new father remove his shirt and hold the baby against his bare chest to promote closeness. Babies adore this and if the father talks or sings, they will turn their focus in the father's direction because they recognize his voice.

In the 1960s, Dr. Frederick Leboyer wrote a book entitled *Birth Without Violence*. He contended that hospital birth was equivalent to an act of violence for the newborn and recommended dimmed lights, hushed voices, delayed umbilical cord clamping, and that the father give the baby a Leboyer bath immediately after birth. The bath, designed to detraumatize birth for the baby by taking him or her from water to water, was simply a small tub filled with warm water in which the father would gently rock the baby back and forth. Steve, who became a father when he was thirty-two, swears that he and his son, Adrian, have such a tight bond because of the Leboyer bath he gave him at birth.

Stand Back, Mother Tiger!

Once you are a new mother you can do a lot to foster your partner's relationship with the baby. Initially it will be tempting for you to be a mother tiger and vigilantly protect your newborn from external forces, including the father. If you can back off from this response and find ways to include him from the very beginning it will strengthen the father-infant bond and make dad feel valued. Fathers are the world's best diaper changers, burpers, bathers, and rockers. Their pinkies are often the perfect size for a stand-in pacifier. They excel at baby massage. If you are breast-feeding, once you are ready to pump your milk and give a bottle, they are wonderful at feeding the baby. If you are bottle-feeding they can share in feeding detail from the beginning.

Essentially, a new father can do everything but breast-feed the baby—and there are those who would if they could! It can really be a struggle for you to allow your partner to take on a specific task. Most often you will feel like you know best or that the baby won't accept nurturing from anybody but you. Unless a man has had a lot of experience with a newborn, he most often will let his partner take the lead and learn from her.

> *Heather had a difficult time allowing her husband, Ed, to take care of the baby. After she had her first baby Heather complained to her mother that Ed wasn't doing things right. He would take the baby in the car and not lock the car door in the backseat; he would let the baby cry too long before picking him up; and he wasn't able to do more than one thing at a time, so if he was home with the baby no housework got done. Her mother's response was, "You have to let Ed figure out his own way of doing things. The only way he will gain confidence is through practice. He might not do it the way you would, but babies are smart—they catch on and understand that one way is mommy's and the other is daddy's." It was very difficult for Heather to let Ed be more involved, but she tried to heed her mother's advice and include him.*

Step Up to the Plate, Dad!

Historically, the role of the father has been to protect his family. Allowing a new dad to follow his instinct to care for his young family is one tradition that is worth preserving. Following the birth of your child, give your partner the opportunity to be the protector of the mother-infant bond. Let him be in charge of crowd control, both in the hospital and at home. Friends and relatives rush to visit a new family and he can keep things calm and organized. When a father takes the initiative to buttress the mother-baby intimacy, he protects and supports the relationship, providing invaluable strength for a new mother.

Let Him Be an Expert

It can be very helpful for a new dad to feel he is the expert at something, say diaper changing, for example. He may become such a specialist that he will show you new methods and short-cuts. If a man has helped raise younger siblings or cousins, and you have had no experience with babies, he may be the one leading the way. It is wonderful when you can learn from each other.

Babysitter Is Not Spelled D-A-D

As a new mother, you might bristle if your partner makes reference to "babysitting" for his new baby. Many new mothers do. Babysitting means being a temporary stand-in for the parent. When two parents are sharing the work of caring for a new baby, neither one of them is the babysitter.

How you negotiate the shared responsibility of the baby is determined by your particular lifestyle and schedule. Each family comes up with a way that works for them. Not all women want their partners to be full participants in the newborn phase. They feel more comfortable sending them back to work, figuring out the baby on their own, and then teaching their partner all the tricks. This might work for some fathers and be upsetting for others who want the hands-on experience from the beginning. It is nearly impossible to anticipate these things before the baby comes. When you are pregnant you may be very independent and feel that you want to do it all on your own. Be aware that once the baby comes you might change your tune.

The most important thing is for you and your partner to discuss your upcoming roles as coparents before the baby comes. Remember that this whole experience is a process and things change continuously. There are so many things you won't know until you get there. Keep the dialogue going for the sake of your relationship and the sake of your baby.

Dads Worksheet

When discussing pregnancy and parenting with my partner, I feel that we:

- ☐ Are able to talk about issues and listen to each other
- ☐ Are able to talk but have trouble listening to each other
- ☐ Have a difficult time communicating
- ☐ Don't talk at all

When my partner feels hurt or jealous in our relationship we:

- ☐ Are able to talk about issues and listen to each other
- ☐ Are able to talk but have trouble listening to each other
- ☐ Have a difficult time communicating
- ☐ Don't talk at all

When we try to make decisions together as a couple we:

- ☐ Are able to talk about issues and listen to each other
- ☐ Are able to talk but have trouble listening to each other
- ☐ Have a difficult time communicating
- ☐ Don't talk at all

I hope that during pregnancy we will be able to:

When I become a mother I expect:

- ☐ To share parenting as much as possible with my partner
- ☐ To ask my partner frequently to do specific things with the baby
- ☐ That I will do most of the child care, but will want his help occasionally
- ☐ That I will cover all the child care while he works
- ☐ To go back to work while he stays home with the baby

The biggest challenges for me in coparenting with my partner will be:

When issues come up for us after the baby is born, I hope we can:

11

Nontraditional Parenting

Though blanket statements about all heterosexual mothers, all lesbian mothers, or all single mothers are rarely illuminating, there are some issues that are undeniably specific to certain populations. The process of conception, the emotional and social aspects of the experience, coming to peace with an identity, and finding acceptance in the community all have a different twist for women living nontraditional lifestyles.

Our traditional concept of motherhood, defined by a woman who carries and gives birth to a baby that is the genetic offspring of her and her partner, is changing before our eyes. Due to amazing advances in medicine, women who would not have been able to become pregnant a generation ago are now having children. Some of these are married women who are unable to conceive, some are single, some are lesbians, and some are surrogates. The path these women take toward conception is certainly more circuitous and varied than the traditional route, with concomitant legal and emotional obstacles to overcome.

Single Mothers

There are a number of routes a single woman might take toward the goal of conception. Some women find themselves pregnant in the absence of a committed partnership and make the decision to raise the child alone. Others are in a relationship with a nonparticipating father. And some single women reach a certain age and decide they want a baby, relationship or not. In order to conceive some of these women arrange for sperm donation from a beloved male friend or use the services of a sperm bank. If they are unable to produce a healthy egg, they may have both sperm and egg donated. Others adopt.

Some single mothers make a commitment to single motherhood and have no interest in a partner; some don't want to be single at all and find themselves in a distressing situation. Others are open to the possibility of having a partner and after entering motherhood alone may find a great one.

> *Three years after her relationship ended Ali was still single. While she didn't want a relationship, she wanted a baby more than ever. So she began investigating sperm banks. Her best friend, Doug, volunteered to be the father. He wanted to father a child, but knew that family life just wasn't for him. She did extensive legal research before making a decision and after weighing all her options, decided that she would take Doug up on his offer. Four months later she became pregnant. Doug was legally the baby's father, but Ali had full custody. This arrangement worked out well for both of them.*

The Importance of Support

Once pregnant, single mothers need a great deal of support, especially when going to doctor's visits and attending prenatal education courses. It makes an enormous difference when a woman has a mother, sister, friend, or other support person to attend both medical visits and classes with her. Ideally, this will be the same person who attends the birth. Sometimes a single mother will hire a doula to provide labor support in addition to having her mother or friend with her. Having a dedicated person available for pregnancy and birth support can give her an extra feeling of security. It will be even more important for a single mother to have several backup plans for when she goes into labor and after the birth. There are also postpartum doulas or baby nurses available in many communities who make home visits after the baby is born.

In many cases a single mother is still in contact with the baby's father during the pregnancy. These situations can bring up a complex set of feelings. She may still love the father and want him to attend prenatal classes with her. On the other hand, he may want to be involved and she may not want him around. It is difficult to know how to best take care of yourself when you are pregnant and in a semicommitted relationship. A woman in this situation may feel a great longing to have the father with her at the birth so they can share the experience. Some hope that having a baby will bring them close enough to overcome the problems of the relationship.

> *Cynthia, a single mother, attended childbirth classes with her best friend, Arlene. The father, Glen, with whom she was still in love, was a man who was significantly older than she and not interested in being a father. He communicated with her intermittently during the pregnancy and she held out hope that the birth of the baby would turn him around. When he did show up to visit, he really wasn't there in spirit and it made her feel even more alone. Her friends, of course, all told her to lose him, but she couldn't let go of wanting to be with him, especially now that she was having his child. When she went into labor, both her friend and childbirth educator went with her to the hospital. They gave her a tremendous amount of support. She called Glen to let him know that she was in labor and hoped that he would show up for the birth. When she was in very active labor, he called the hospital. She waited and waited for him, but he never came. Her expectations were unrealistic, but she was vulnerable. Her emotional state impacted her ability to focus on her labor and take care of herself.*

A single mother might feel even more isolated and fearful as she takes the leap into the strange and wonderful world of motherhood because she is flying solo. Hopefully for the first several weeks, a relative, friend, or hired professional will stay and help with the baby. Again, if the father is standing in the wings, it can create a lot of confusion for a new mother and intensify her stress.

Creativity Is Key

Creativity is a great asset for single moms when organizing support for their child. Some women have a close male friend in their lives who becomes a father figure. Some women find other single mothers to align themselves with and either live together as a community or share child care. Communal living with children makes sense—single women who share the responsibility and strain of child rearing may be less stressed than their married counterparts who live isolated lives. Other women live with their parents or close to them and the grandparents assume an active role in the upbringing of the child. This is a great gift for the loving grandparents, grandchild, and mother. Women who have the space and the financial means, especially busy professional women, might hire a live-in nanny.

Lesbian Mothers

Lesbian mothers often go through much more preconception planning than their heterosexual counterparts. For the most part they use sperm donors to become pregnant, though some self-inseminate using a friend's sperm and a turkey baster. There are advantages and disadvantages to using a known (directed) versus an anonymous (program) donor.

Directed Donors

The up side, if all goes well with a known donor, is that the mothers and the child have the advantage of knowing the biological father. In addition, if the insemination is done with a doctor as the go-between, or the woman self-inseminates at home, the sperm is fresh, so chances of becoming pregnant may be better. You may need to look for a doctor who will perform this service. Because the sperm is not tested over time, there is a risk that it may be infected with HIV, hepatitis B or C, or another sexually transmitted disease.

> *To provide a biological link, Heather and her partner, Nancy, chose to use Nancy's brother, Hank, as the sperm donor. Once Hank agreed Nancy became concerned about using fresh sperm because it would not have been thoroughly screened. However, she did not want to wait the six months it would take to have the sperm frozen and to have Hank retested. This presented a dilemma for them as a couple.*

In terms of legal concerns, even if a preinsemination contract is drawn up without a doctor performing the insemination, the father could still contest custody and may even succeed in gaining it. Many women who use a known donor do so under the guidance of a physician, which establishes legal intention. Once sperm is given to a licensed physician, a father relinquishes any legal parentage.

Program Donors

Sperm bank sperm is carefully screened multiple times for HIV, hepatitis B and C, syphilis, and other sexually transmitted diseases. In addition, it is screened for Tay-Sachs, sickle cell anemia, and cystic fibrosis if the donor is at risk for any of these genetic diseases. The sperm is frozen and quarantined for a six-month period, after which the donors are retested and the sperm is released. Because of the length of the screening process, fresh sperm cannot be used. Women have access to thorough medical records of family health and genetic history going back to the grandparents' generation, and the opportunity to choose from a number of candidates. This option is certainly more expensive than self-insemination (it can cost as much as $200 per sperm sample), but it does have the advantage of several inherent safeguards. With donor insemination, it is unlikely that the child will be able to meet the biological father, and this father also cannot sue for custody. Sperm can be reserved in advance through a sperm bank. There is typically a limit to how many births each donor can facilitate.

For a lesbian wanting to become pregnant, finding an open-minded doctor who will inseminate her can often be the greatest obstacle. It can also feel risky for a woman to come out if she is living in a sheltered community. A woman living in San Francisco, for example, will have more options than a woman in a small town. Women can undergo a great deal of soul-searching in preparation for insemination. Here is how Anna describes the process of deciding to become pregnant.

> I would say that much of what I went through is not related to being gay. However, from my point of view it is hard to separate it out. I know that I was looking for a partner because my clock was ticking. I had a lot of work to do to get up the guts to get pregnant, and part of that was talking my partner, Ellen, into it. Also talking myself into it, and getting past all the guilt trips about being selfish. I was asking myself if I

should adopt, if it is okay to bring children into an alternative
family, and would I be able to pull it off. I thought about
everything for many months, and in great detail. I knew this
was the most important decision for my life. I took a long time
to research the alternatives and I talked to everyone I knew
who had kids, or was thinking about having kids, especially
my family. I had to have their support.

Becoming pregnant using donor sperm can take a lot of time.
Everything has to be timed perfectly and even then conception
doesn't always occur. It can be frustrating for both partners and
draining, both financially and emotionally. Some couples go
through this with more ease than others.

Lynda and Maggie decided they wanted to go the sperm bank
route. Maggie, at age thirty-seven, was given pergonal, a fer-
tility enhancing medication, but was unable to conceive with
the first donor. She switched donors and had two miscarriages.
At age forty-one she decided to try one more time, but this
time with a known donor. They found Matthew, a married
man, and worked with a lawyer to draw up all the necessary
legal papers. Though it was a known donor, they did the
insemination under the guidance of a doctor. It worked the
first time. Originally they had a list of specifics they were look-
ing for—certain physical traits, intellect, religion, and health,
but as their search progressed, they began letting go of precon-
ceived notions and focused on finding a man they felt good
about. Four months after Maggie conceived, Matthew's wife,
Melissa, became pregnant. Matthew would now have two chil-
dren in the same community, five months apart in age. After
the birth of their son Joshua, Lynda said that selecting the
donor was the hardest part. They were aware they would have
a lifelong relationship with this man.

Who exactly are these sperm donors? College kids needing
to make a few extra bucks who would rather give sperm than
blood? Gay men who know they won't have children of their own
but want to contribute to the next generation? Men who love children but due to personal circumstances won't have any of their
own? As sperm bank children grow older, some of them want to
know who their father is and have the chance to meet any half-
brothers or -sisters they might have. Some sperm banks have an

ID release program, whereby donors agree to meet their children at age eighteen; others have reunions where children of the same donor can meet each other.

Peeling Back Layer after Layer

Tamar and Leila thought about having a baby for two years before Leila conceived. They began with a vision of the ideal donor and along the way had to modify their picture. Tamar describes the experience they had been through as peeling back layer after layer, and in the process having to let go of their dream vision.

Tamar and her partner, Leila, felt overwhelmed by the process they had to go through to become pregnant. Once they decided, it took almost two years to gather all their resources, find an attorney, put all the legal pieces in place, find a physician, and finally, locate a donor who met their specifications. To begin with, Tamar had to go through the grief of not being able to make a baby with the person she loved. Then with each step they had to let go of expectations and accept that reality wouldn't always match their ideal. Tamar is Caucasian and Leila is Chinese. They wanted their baby to reflect this mix. They found a known donor for Leila, who was introduced through a good friend. The donor, Stephan, was a highly creative gay man who didn't want to be a father, but saw this as the ultimate act of creativity. They used the services of a medical clinic for a supervised fresh semen transfer. The sperm bank did a donor screening test. Their attorney drew up a business contract and they paid the donor, creating a legal, binding contract. Leila became pregnant after six inseminations. Tamar and Leila had planned all along to have two children. When their daughter was two, they began researching a donor for Tamar. It was far more difficult to find a Chinese donor than it had been to find a Caucasian donor. Once they located a donor and began inseminations, Tamar discovered that she had fertility problems. After a great deal of soul-searching, they decided that Leila would have the second child. They used Stephan's sperm again, though this time they did it on their own at home and it took three inseminations.

Will the Real Birth Mother Please Stand Up?

A big question that might arise is, "Which one of us is going to carry the baby?" It is often the case that one partner has the strong desire to become pregnant while the other doesn't, so she becomes the birth mother. During the course of time, these feelings and desires can certainly change. If both partners are able to conceive, a number of options are available.

Yvonne and Dierdre had been together for more than seven years. When Yvonne turned thirty-five the tick of her biological clock was unrelenting. They had never discussed having a baby; it had not been part of their life plan. Yvonne had thought about it intermittently over the years, but never felt compelled to take any further steps. Dierdre had never had a desire to be pregnant. Knowing this would amount to a huge change in their lifestyle, they talked for months before making the decision to start researching sperm banks. Six months later, Dierdre was inseminated for the first time. It took three tries for her to become pregnant.

Cheryl and Monica both wanted babies at the same time. They were both inseminated by different donors and both became pregnant. They were often seen in their community tooling down the street with both their babies, who were a month apart in age, in their strollers.

Jayne and Suzanna decided to have a baby. Suzanna was the one who wanted to be pregnant and was inseminated with donor sperm. Looking toward the future, they reserved sperm from the same donor, in the event that Suzanna might carry another child. When their child turned two, Jayne decided that she too wanted to experience pregnancy. Jayne was inseminated with the sperm they had reserved, so now their babies would have the same father.

When Violet became pregnant using a sperm donor, she and her partner, Sue, had made the decision to have only one child. Four years later, Sue wanted to have a baby. They tried to see if they could secure sperm from the same donor but were unsuccessful. So, they used the same sperm bank, but Sue became pregnant with another donor's sperm.

Who's Called Mommy?

Interesting questions arise once the baby is born. What do children call their mothers when they have two? Some mothers encourage the child to use two different names such as "mama" and "mommy," or "Mommy Jill" and "Mommy Susan." Babies growing up with two mothers are pretty clear about who is who. Do they have a different bond with the mother who carries them through pregnancy and breast-feeds them than the mother who doesn't? Is the mother who carries the baby more bonded to the baby than the mother who doesn't? What are the advantages of having two mothers? What are the disadvantages? What kind of support is available for mothers and children?

Once their son Daniel was born, Donna, who had carried the pregnancy, was of course the one who breast-fed him. She adored her son, but unlike her partner Simone, she was not a terribly affectionate person. Simone, though not the birth mother, had a much more hands-on relationship with the baby. They both felt a strong maternal connection with their son, though they expressed it in different ways.

Once pregnancy has been achieved, the thing that can be tricky for lesbian couples is that though only one of them is pregnant, both of them are women and mothers. The bond that is recognized in society is the bond of the birth mother and baby, so the nonbirth mother can potentially end up feeling invalidated or invisible.

When Helen and Elaine attended their first meeting of their childbirth class, they participated in an exercise in which the couples were split up into two groups: the women and the partners. Elaine, who was pregnant, went with the women; Helen went with the fathers and felt out of place. In talking with Elaine later that evening, Helen realized, had she been with the pregnant women, she still would have felt awkward. Following the third class, she stayed to speak with the childbirth educator and found it beneficial just to air her feelings. She really felt like she didn't belong anywhere. Also, she had been concerned that the instructor was feeling uncomfortable having them in the class with all the other couples being heterosexual, or that other couples were ill at ease. Helen had hoped there would be other lesbian couples in the class.

Find Your Comfort Zone

It would have been advantageous had Helen called the educator before the class to gather information about her philosophy and approach to teaching. It isn't always clear in advance what issues will arise in a classroom setting, but had Helen explained her situation and gotten feedback from the instructor, she would have been more prepared for the level of support that would be available. Childbirth educators tend to be compassionate people and want students to feel at home and comfortable in their classes. In general, they try to be very inclusive and will use the word "partner" or "coach," rather than "husband," to refer to the support person attending class with the pregnant woman. It also helps the educator tremendously if she has advance information about the mix of students she will be working with and if there will be special needs to address.

Some communities have prenatal classes designed especially for single and lesbian mothers. For some lesbian couples it might feel more comfortable to attend a specialized class; others have no problem with or prefer a more eclectic class. In certain devout communities it is normal for women to attend childbirth classes alone or with another woman. Among Orthodox Jews, for example, men do not attend the classes or the birth.

The amount of external support a woman receives will depend on the disposition of her family members and her community. Her family, neighbors, church, or synagogue may receive her with open arms or she may be regarded as an outsider by those who live more proscribed lives. Of course this can be true for anyone who lives a less than traditional lifestyle. Certainly, lesbian mothers have different concerns than single mothers with regard to issues of acceptance.

When Barb became pregnant, things changed. People in the grocery store started talking to her about her pregnancy and every so often someone would ask about the baby's father. When she and Kyla were out together it was not assumed that they were partners and Kyla started to feel invisible. Once Micah was born their own community showered them with support and acceptance. But when they went into the community at large more questions about his father arose. Barb and Kyla realized what an insular life they had been leading and were unprepared for these responses.

Legal Realities

For a lesbian couple living where they are unable to marry, having a baby becomes the legal link for them, and also validates the relationship in the eyes of grandparents and the community. A family is a much more accepted social unit than two women living together as a couple. Some parents who have been unable to condone a daughter's lifestyle, possibly to the point of complete alienation, find tolerance and even acceptance once a grandchild enters the picture.

When two women have a baby together the nonbirth mother is not considered a legal parent. Second parent adoption is, so far, the most widely used legal procedure for the nonbirth mothers. This requires a great deal of paperwork, involves social services, and takes time. The increasing number of sperm bank and egg donor babies has initiated a new wave of legal responses. There have been some cases in which legal parenthood has been established prior to the baby's birth so that adoption is not necessary. The Uniform Parentage Act is a law that was adopted by the state of California among others. When a couple files a petition under it, it is filed jointly by both parents, and argues that intention more than anything is what establishes parentage.

Surrogate Mothers

Surrogate mothers face very different issues than either single or lesbian mothers because they become pregnant with no intention of keeping the baby. In reality there are two mothers involved in this type of pregnancy: the mother who carries the baby and gives birth and the mother who parents the child. In some cases these two mothers have a legal partnership only; in others they also have a personal relationship.

Some women are unable to carry a baby because they have an abnormal uterus, no uterus, no egg production, or a health problem that prevents them from sustaining a pregnancy. In some of these cases a woman or couple will seek out a surrogate mother. Some people go through agencies; others choose a friend or relative to carry a baby for them. The surrogate mother can be a rented womb, meaning sperm and egg of the couple are inserted into her uterus, or if the woman has no eggs, the surrogate may supply both donor egg and womb. Similar to an open adoption, in the case of a surrogate the parents often provide financial support during the pregnancy on top of a designated fee for carrying the baby. The parents are likely to attend birth classes with the surrogate mother and be present at the birth of the baby. Depending on the desires of the parents, the surrogate mother may be invited to stay in touch with the child and participate in family events. It goes without saying that extensive legal documents are drawn up in these situations.

Who are the women who become surrogate mothers? They range from women who have never had a child to mothers who want to share the gift of motherhood with those unable to carry a baby.

Judith and her husband could not afford to have any more children, but Judith loved being pregnant and wanted to experience it at least one more time. She also felt that if she could carry a baby for another woman it would be the greatest gift she could ever give. She met with a doctor in Los Angeles who matched women with surrogate mothers. She was matched with a woman on the East Coast in her forties and was paid $10,000 for carrying the baby. The "adoptive" couple came out to California to be present for the birth of their child. Judith enjoyed the experience so much that three years later she carried a baby for another woman.

Sophie and Bob, who were both musicians, had been married for four years when they began trying to conceive. After a year of trying and extensive fertility testing and treatment, Sophie was told she could not become pregnant. They considered adopting a child or finding a surrogate. After much soul-searching and discussion they decided to adopt. Their close friend Jackie, who was a lesbian, offered to carry the baby for them. She very much wanted to experience pregnancy and childbirth but didn't want to have a family. The arrangement was wonderful for all of them. Though Jackie had never wanted to have children, she thoroughly enjoyed being pregnant. They lived in the same city so they were all able to share both the challenges and the excitement. When the baby was born Sophie was the "main mom," but Jackie spent a lot of time with her, particularly when Sophie and Bob went out on the road with their band. All three sets of grandparents fell in love with their new granddaughter. In a sense they formed their own parenting commune, able to shower their daughter with so much love.

Motherhood in the Twenty-first Century

With modern scientific advances being what they are, the barriers that used to stand in a woman's way, blocking her path toward motherhood are dissolving. Because a woman is not able to become pregnant does not mean she won't become a mother. Women who have adopted children have shown that you don't have to give birth to a child in order to be a mother to him or her, that pregnancy and mothering are two separate experiences. Certainly with ever-increasing options, come ever-increasing legal and emotional hurdles women will need to overcome.

We have yet to see how the new identity and familial structures that children face will be played out. It is interesting to imagine the dialogue that will take place among them: "Hi, I am the child of sperm donor number 218 and the half-sibling of his two other donor children. Who's your dad?" "My first mother was pregnant with me, but my second mother raised me." "I have two mommies, one breast-fed me, the other didn't." We have begun a new chapter in family life and dynamics.

Nontraditional Parenting Worksheet

When I think about the options for motherhood that are available to me, I feel:

When I consider my choice to have a nontraditional family, I feel:

I plan to use a:

☐ known donor

☐ program donor

The advantages of choosing a known donor are:

The advantages of choosing a program donor are:

The disadvantages of choosing a known donor are:

The disadvantages of choosing a program donor are:

When I think about becoming pregnant and how I will be received by my family and community, I feel:

When I consider all the legal and practical issues that are ahead of me, I feel:

Conclusion

After all the discussion of swelling bellies, hormonal roller coasters, five P.M. bathrobe days, and sleep deprived nights, are you starting to see motherhood in a new light? Are you ready to let go of the idealized image you may have had of yourself as a mother? Are you prepared to accept that once you have a baby you may have some, but not all of the answers and that you will be challenged to take each phase as it comes?

Your inner voice may be calling out, "No, not me. I'm not prepared for all of this!" Or it may be saying, "Okay, it's not all under my control, let's roll the dice." Or maybe, "Well, on the one hand I kind of feel ready, but on the other hand . . . I'm just not sure." The truth is that 75 percent prepared might be as ready as you will ever feel.

Despite the fears, anxieties, and ambivalence; despite the lifestyle upheaval and identity shifts; despite the physical challenges, most new mothers say that by the time their baby is two-months old they can't remember what life was like before, and that they have no idea what it was they used to do with their time. Pregnancy is the first step, the door that leads you to a new and ever-expanding space in your life and your heart, toward a love that is impossible to fully understand in advance. Once your baby is in your arms, it will all fall into place; the understanding will come, much like a light suddenly being switched on.

There is no one way to make the pregnancy decision. It is a unique experience for each of us. In thinking about it, continue to gather knowledge, stay flexible, and trust your instincts.

Whether you want to stay in the "thinking pregnant" phase just a bit longer or move into the "becoming pregnant" phase, recognize that becoming pregnant is one of many new beginnings you will experience in your life. In the meantime make the most of this time with yourself, your partner, your friends, and your family before embarking on this life-altering journey. A day will come when discussions about this chapter of your life will begin with the words, "Remember when . . ."

Appendix

Though some of the information, solicited or not, that you receive about pregnancy, childbirth, and motherhood is sound, without a doubt some misinformation will also make its way to you. How will you sift through the barrage of opinions and advice that you encounter as you prepare for pregnancy? Here are some of the more common myths and realities you might come across:

I will need to eat for two when I'm pregnant.
Myth. True, your caloric intake will increase, but two servings of everything? No, thank you.

I will gain an enormous amount of weight when I'm pregnant.
This is not at all necessary.

Once I become a new mother I will have a permanent glow and everything will be organized.
Hmmm. Solid organization can take some months to achieve and for some mothers varying degrees of chaos remain a constant. Permaglow is an ideal, not a reality.

My personality will change drastically once I become a mother.
Absolutely. You will resemble a mother tiger. Even women who have never raised their voice will raise the roof over anything, animate or inanimate, that could conceivably threaten their child. The concern for your child's safety takes over.

Once I am a mother I will feel a kind of love I have never felt before.
Women report feeling so much love for their baby that it hurts. The intensity of maternal love comes as a surprise to most

women. Moments of ecstasy, gratitude, and wonder can, at times, feel overwhelming.

I will bounce back right after the birth of my baby.
Some women get their bodies back and feel full of energy sooner than others. It is more common for a woman to feel she is in a time and energy vortex for a minimum of two months. For some it takes literally years to recover from the effects of the pregnancy, birth, and sleep deprivation.

My clothes will never fit me again.
When you are pregnant and hold up your normal bra, panties, or jeans, they resemble doll clothes. It is unimaginable that they will ever fit again. Some women are back in their jeans by six weeks postpartum; others take many months or even years to lose their baby weight. Women's bodies are different, so not surprisingly they differ in the way they respond to child bearing. Exercise and diet play an essential part in maintaining a healthy weight.

My body will never be the same.
Pretty much irrefutable. You've never had a baby grow inside you before, have you? Some women's bodies don't change much after childbirth. Other women's breasts change shape and size and their hips broaden. There are women who experience less visible effects such as stretch marks, varicose veins, and urinary incontinence. Some women have a new, improved body after giving birth because they begin to exercise and take care of themselves for the first time.

My breasts will never be the same.
The key word here is "genes." Some women's breasts grow dramatically in pregnancy, for example from a 32A to a 36D. Some women grow just a bit. The more your breasts change, the more likelihood there will be of getting stretch marks if you are genetically predisposed to them.

If I rub oil on my tummy religiously each day I won't get stretch marks.
If you are genetically predisposed to having stretch marks, there is not much you can do to avoid them. Oiling your tummy will keep the skin from being dry, but won't stop stretch marks from occurring. If you do get them, they will fade over time.

Breastfeeding is going to be a breeze, it will naturally fall into place.
For a select few, breastfeeding falls easily into place. But in general, new mothers are surprised by the amount of effort that goes into breastfeeding a baby. They are unprepared for being engorged when the milk comes in and for the nipple soreness they experience. It can take some time to get a baby to properly latch on. Once a new mom gets past the first three weeks, discomfort is typically resolved and then breastfeeding becomes not only a breeze, but a very fulfilling experience.

If I breast-feed I won't need to use birth control.
For about 98 percent of the women who breast-feed exclusively this proves an effective method of birth control for up to six months. This is because full-time breastfeeding suppresses ovulation. Be aware that if you begin using a breast pump the contraceptive effects of breastfeeding become unreliable. Also, you can begin ovulating as early as six weeks postpartum, so it is wise to use a form of birth control when resuming intercourse if you aren't planning another pregnancy right away.

When I think about my baby, my milk will be released and leak all over my shirt.
For the majority of women this is true. Nursing pads, placed in your bra to soak up the extra milk, can be a great help for a breastfeeding mother.

I will never have sex again.
A bit of an exaggeration, though it depends what you mean by "again." Some women are ready right away. It may take you weeks, even months to feel comfortable with sex. Many women have decreased sexual desire while breastfeeding.

Having a baby will enhance my relationship with my partner.
Even with the stress and loss of sleep, for many couples a new baby brings them closer together and enriches their relationship.

I will never sleep through the night again and will be a zombie for life.
There is that rare baby who sleeps through the night at six weeks, but most take at least three to six months, if not much longer, to establish a consistent sleep-through-the-night routine. This sleepless phase has been described as brutal by new mothers, mostly because of the cumulative effects of sleep deprivation.

Understand that once the newborn period ends, you will continue to have phases of sleeplessness in your life as your child grows and develops.

The exhaustion factor won't be so bad.
This is true for some women either because they have a baby who is a good sleeper from the outset or they are able to withstand sleep deprivation.

I will never have the luxury of reading a newspaper article, much less an entire book again.
It may be six months before you can become engrossed in a book or article again. Be prepared to feel extremely tired and unable to concentrate.

I will be unable to watch the evening news for months.
This is true for many new moms. The subject matter and images on the news are often too violent and distressing for new mothers who are emotionally sensitive and don't have the ability to detach, which is required when viewing upsetting images.

I will become sentimental and have no control over my tear ducts.
Don't count on being able to sit through Hallmark commercials dry-eyed.

I will not go to the bathroom alone again for years.
For the most part, you will have a devoted companion in the bathroom with you. Children don't value privacy the way adults do.

I will worry obsessively about my child's well-being for the rest of my life.
An intrinsic part of being a parent is being a worry wart. Some mothers take worrying to its ultimate and become catastrophizers. There are so many things to be concerned about with a baby that it is nearly impossible to avoid worry. What you can control is the degree to which you let the fear overtake your life and relationship with your child.

I will never be able to leave my baby and go back to work.
For some women this is true. Leaving their infant in the care of another person while they work is simply too much to bear.

Returning to work and leaving my baby in child care will be fine.
Again, for some women this is true. They enjoy resuming a professional life and feel able to balance motherhood and work.

Independent women do not become overly attached to their babies.
Not many new mothers, independent or otherwise, can pull this one off.

All of my friends without children will abandon me.
This may happen with some of your nonparent friends, but certainly not with all of them.

I will make a whole new group of "mommy friends."
This is a wonderful and exciting reality.

I am never going to let my child control my life.
Please share your secret for managing this with the rest of us.

I will become just like my mother.
As you mother your new baby you may begin to hear the familiar ring of your mother's voice in your head. This strikes a note of terror in the hearts of some new mothers, but others find it reassuring. Certainly your response will depend upon how you feel about your mother and the nature of your relationship with her.

I am going to repeat all the mistakes my parents made.
Given that you are a woman who is "thinking pregnant," rather than blindly falling into pregnancy and motherhood, you are already laying the groundwork for being a conscious parent. You are not in any way required or doomed to repeat the missteps of your parents.

My life will never be the same.
Bravo! You have assimilated the central theme of this book.

References

Adashek J.A., A.M. Peaceman, J.A. Lopez-Zeno, J.P. Minogue, and M.L. Socol. 1993. Factors contributing to the increased cesarean birth rate in older parturient women. *American Journal of Obstetrics & Gynecology* 169(4):936-40.

Agarwal, S.K., and A.F. Haney. 1994. Does recommending timed intercourse really help the infertile couple? *Obstetrics & Gynecology* 84(2):307-10.

Alberman, E. 1987. Maternal age and spontaneous abortion. In *Spontaneous and Recurrent Abortion*, edited by M.J. Bennett and D.K. Edmonds. Oxford: Blackwell Scientific Publications.

American Academy of Pediatrics. 1997. Breastfeeding and the use of human milk. *Pediatrics* 100(6):1035-39.

American Academy of Pediatrics. 2000. Changing concepts of Sudden Infant Death Syndrome: Implications for infant sleeping environment and sleep position (RE9946). *Pediatrics* 105(3):650-56.

American Academy of Pediatrics. 1999. Circumcision policy statement. *Pediatrics* 103(3):686-93.

Artal, R., and C. Sherman. 1999. Exercise during pregnancy. *The Physician and Sports Medicine* 27(8).

Carson S.A. 1995. Management of early pregnancy and pregnancy outcome in assisted reproductive technologies. In *Infertility*, edited by W.R. Keye, R.J. Chang, R.W. Rebor and M.R. Soules. Philadelphia: WB. Saunders.

Daviaud, J., D. Fournet, C. Bollongue, G.P. Guilliem, A. Leblanc, C. Casellas, and B. Pau. 1993. Reliability and feasibility of pregnancy home-use test: Laboratory validation and diagnostic evaluation by 638 volunteers. *Clinical Chemistry* 39(1):7-8.

Dewey, K., M. Heinig, and L. Nomnsen-Rivers. 1995, Differences in morbidity between breastfed and formula fed infants. 126(5):696-702.

Ebrahim, S.H., S.T. Diekman, R.L Floyd, and P. Decoufle. 1999. Rise in binge drinking during pregnancy. *American Journal of Obstetrics & Gynecology* 180:1-7.

Enger, S.M., R.K. Ross, A. Paganini-Hill, and L. Bernstein. 1998. Breastfeeding experience and breast cancer risk among post-menopausal women. *Cancer, Epidemiology, Biomarkers & Prevention* 7(5):365-69.

Fretts R.C., J. Schmittdiel, F.H. McLean, R.H. Usher, and M.B. Goldman. 1995. Increased maternal age and the risk of fetal death. *New England Journal of Medicine* 333(15):1002-4.

Gabbe, G., J. Niebyl, and J. Simpson. 1991. *Obstetrics Normal & Problem Pregnancies*, 2nd edition. Livingstone, New York: Churchill.

Guttmacher A.F. 1956. Factors affecting normal expectancy of conception. *Journal of American Medical Association* 161:855-60.

Gwinn, M.L., N.C. Lee, P.H. Rhodes, and P.M. Layde. 1990. Pregnancy, breastfeeding, and oral contraceptives and the risk of epithelial ovarian cancer. *Journal of Clinical Epidemiology* 43(6):55-68.

Haustein, K.O. 1999. Cigarette smoking, nicotine and pregnancy. *Journal of Clinical Pharmacological Therapy* 37(9):417-27.

The Health Benefits of Smoking Cessation. 1990. A Report of the Surgeon General. U.S. Department of Health and Human Services. DHHS Publication No. (CDC) 90-8416.

Hung T.H., W.Y. Shau, C.C. Hsieh, T.H. Chiu, J.J. Hsu, and T.T. Hseih. 1999. Risk factors for placenta accretia. *Obstetrics & Gynecology* 93(4):545-5.

King, H. 1998. Epidemiology of glucose intolerance and gestational diabetes in women of childbearing age. *Diabetes Care* Suppl 2:B9-13.

Klaus, M., J. Kennell, and P. Klaus. 1993. *Mothering the Mother*. Cambridge: Perseus Books.

Kramer, F.M., A.J Stunkard, K.A. Marshall, S. McKinney, and J. Liebshutz. 1993. Breastfeeding reduces maternal lower-body fat. *Journal of American Diet Association* 93(4):429-33.

National Academy of Sciences. 1989. *Recommended Dietary Allowances*, 10th edition. Washington DC: National Academy Press.

Resultan, E. 1999. Getting moms to quit. *Healthplan* 40(1):17-22.

Scheibmeir, M., and K. O'Connell. 1997. In harm's way: Childbearing women and nicotine. *Journal of Obstetrics Gynecology and Neonatal Nursing* 26(4):477-84.

Schwartz, D., and M.J. Mayaux. 1982. Female fecundity as a function of age: Results of artificial insemination in 2193 nulliparous women with azospermic husbands. *New England Journal of Medicine* 307:404-06.

Society for Assisted Reproductive Technology, The American Society of Reproductive Medicine. 1999. Assisted reproductive technology in the United States: 1996 results. *Fertility & Sterility*. 71(5):798-807.

Steiner, M. 1998. Perinatal mood disorders. *Psychopharmacology Bulletin* 34(3):301-306.

Terp, I.M., and P.B. Mortensen. 1998. Post-partum psychoses: Clinical diagnoses and relative risk of admission after parturition. *The British Journal of Psychiatry* 172(6):521-526.

Vercellini, P., G. Zuliani, M.T. Rognoni, L. Trespidi, S. Oldani, and A. Cardinale. 1993. Pregnancy at forty and over: A case-control study. *European Journal of Obstetric & Gynecological Reproductive Biology* 48(3):191-5.

Vermesh, M., O.A. Kletzky, and V. Davajan. 1987. Monitoring techniques to predict ovulation, *Fertility & Sterility* 46:259.

Von Hertzen, H. 1999. WHO calls breastfeeding an effective birth control method. *Fetility & Sterility* 72:431-444.

Weissman, M.M., V. Warner, P.J. Wickramaratne, and D.B. Kandel. 1999. Maternal smoking increases the long-term risk of behavioral problems in boys and in girls. *Journal of the American Academy of Child and Adolescent Psychiatry* 38:892-99.

World Health Organization. 1985. Appropriate technology for birth. *Lancet*: 436-7.

http://www.babycenter.com/calculator/7060.html.

http://www.census.gov/prod/2000pubs/c25-0004.pdf.

http://www.dol.gov/dol/esa/public/regs/statutes/whd/fmla.htm.

http://www.family internet.com/pregcom/05040150.htm.

http://www.march-of-dimes.org/Programs2/FolicAcid/perifaxartic le.htm

http://www.parentsplace.com/fertility/contraception/qa/ 0,3105,13049,00.html.

Resources

Baby Care

Klaus, Marshall and Phyllis. 1998. *Your Amazing Newborn.* Cambridge: Perseus Books.

Leboyer, Frederick. 1978. *Birth Without Violence.* New York: Alfred A. Knopf.

Sears, William. 1993. *The Baby Book.* Boston: Little, Brown & Co.

Breastfeeding

Huggins, Kathleen. 1995. *The Nursing Mother's Companion.* Boston: Harvard Common Press.

La Leche League. 1991. *The Womanly Art of Breastfeeding.* New York: Penguin.

Parenting

Brazelton, T. Berry, M.D. 1994. *Touchpoints: Your Child's Emotional and Behavioral Development.* Reading, Mass.: Perseus Books.

Brott, Armin, and Jennifer Ash. 1995. *The Expectant Father: Facts, Tips, and Advice for Dads-to-Be.* New York: Abbeville Press.

Kabat-Zinn, John, and Myla Kabat. 1998. *Everyday Blessings: The Inner Work of Mindful Parenting.* New York: Hyperion.

Pregnancy & Childbirth

Balaskas, Janet. 1994. *Preparing for Birth with Yoga: Exercises for Pregnancy and Childbirth*. Boston: Element.

Bradley Robert. 1981. *Husband Coached Childbirth*. New York: Harper & Row.

Flanagan, G. 1996. *Beginning Life: The Marvelous Journey from Conception to Birth*. London: Dorling Kindersley.

Kitzinger, Sheila. 1980. *The Complete Book of Pregnancy & Childbirth*. New York: Alfred A. Knopf.333

Klaus, Marshall, John Kennell, and Phyllis Klaus. 1993. *Mothering the Mother*. Cambridge: Perseus Books.

Nilsson, Lennart. 1990. *A Child Is Born*. New York: Delacorte Press.

Nilsson, Lennart. 1986. *The Miracle of Life*. Swedish Television Corporation. (video cassette)

Sears, William. 1997. *The Pregnancy Book*. Boston: Little, Brown & Co.

Sears, William. 1994. *The Birth Book*. Boston: Little, Brown & Co.

Simkin, Penny. 1989. *The Birth Partner*. Boston: The Harvard Common Press.

Simkin, Penny, Janet Whally, and Ann Keppler. 1991. *Pregnancy Childbirth and the Newborn: A Complete Guide for Expectant Parents*. New York: Meadowbrook.

Steelman, Megan V. 1994. *The Relaxation Rhythm: Pregnancy*. Los Angeles: Vered Production. (audio cassette)

Fertility

Jarrett, John C. II, and Deidra T. Rausch. 1998. *The Fertility Guide: A Couples Handbook for When You Want to Have a Baby (More Than Anything Else)*. Santa Fe, N.M.: Health Press.

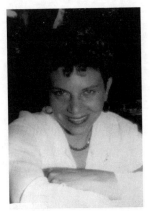

Megan Steelman is the Director of Perinatal Education and the Breastfeeding Center at Kaiser Permanente in San Francisco, California. The codesigner of Body in Balance, an annual series of workshops on women's health, Ms. Steelman lives in Berkeley, California with her daughter Austyn and son Laine.

(Author photo by George Hall)

Some Other New Harbinger Self-Help Titles

Family Guide to Emotional Wellness, $24.95
Undefended Love, $13.95
The Great Big Book of Hope, $15.95
Don't Leave it to Chance, $13.95
Emotional Claustrophobia, $12.95
The Relaxation & Stress Reduction Workbook, Fifth Edition, $19.95
The Loneliness Workbook, $14.95
Thriving with Your Autoimmune Disorder, $16.95
Illness and the Art of Creative Self-Expression, $13.95
The Interstitial Cystitis Survival Guide, $14.95
Outbreak Alert, $15.95
Don't Let Your Mind Stunt Your Growth, $10.95
Energy Tapping, $14.95
Under Her Wing, $13.95
Self-Esteem, Third Edition, $15.95
Women's Sexualitites, $15.95
Knee Pain, $14.95
Helping Your Anxious Child, $12.95
Breaking the Bonds of Irritable Bowel Syndrome, $14.95
Multiple Chemical Sensitivity: A Survival Guide, $16.95
Dancing Naked, $14.95
Why Are We Still Fighting, $15.95
From Sabotage to Success, $14.95
Parkinson's Disease and the Art of Moving, $15.95
A Survivor's Guide to Breast Cancer, $13.95
Men, Women, and Prostate Cancer, $15.95
Make Every Session Count: Getting the Most Out of Your Brief Therapy, $10.95
Virtual Addiction, $12.95
After the Breakup, $13.95
Why Can't I Be the Parent I Want to Be?, $12.95
The Secret Message of Shame, $13.95
The OCD Workbook, $18.95
Tapping Your Inner Strength, $13.95
Binge No More, $14.95
When to Forgive, $12.95
Practical Dreaming, $12.95
Healthy Baby, Toxic World, $15.95
Making Hope Happen, $14.95
I'll Take Care of You, $12.95
Survivor Guilt, $14.95
Children Changed by Trauma, $13.95
Understanding Your Child's Sexual Behavior, $12.95
The Self-Esteem Companion, $10.95
The Gay and Lesbian Self-Esteem Book, $13.95
Making the Big Move, $13.95
How to Survive and Thrive in an Empty Nest, $13.95
Living Well with a Hidden Disability, $15.95
Overcoming Repetitive Motion Injuries the Rossiter Way, $15.95
What to Tell the Kids About Your Divorce, $13.95
The Divorce Book, Second Edition, $15.95
Claiming Your Creative Self: True Stories from the Everyday Lives of Women, $15.95
Taking Control of TMJ, $13.95
Winning Against Relapse: A Workbook of Action Plans for Recurring Health and Emotional Problems, $14.95
Facing 30: Women Talk About Constructing a Real Life and Other Scary Rites of Passage, $12.95
The Worry Control Workbook, $15.95
Wanting What You Have: A Self-Discovery Workbook, $18.95
When Perfect Isn't Good Enough: Strategies for Coping with Perfectionism, $13.95
Earning Your Own Respect: A Handbook of Personal Responsibility, $12.95
High on Stress: A Woman's Guide to Optimizing the Stress in Her Life, $13.95
Infidelity: A Survival Guide, $13.95
Stop Walking on Eggshells, $14.95
Consumer's Guide to Psychiatric Drugs, $16.95
The Fibromyalgia Advocate: Getting the Support You Need to Cope with Fibromyalgia and Myofascial Pain, $18.95
Working Anger: Preventing and Resolving Conflict on the Job, $12.95
Healthy Living with Diabetes, $13.95
Better Boundries: Owning and Treasuring Your Life, $13.95
Goodbye Good Girl, $12.95
Fibromyalgia & Chronic Myofascial Pain Syndrome, $19.95
The Depression Workbook: Living With Depression and Manic Depression, $17.95